HOW TO COPE WITH STRESS

Overcoming Common Problems

HOW TO COPE
WITH STRESS

Dr Peter Tyrer
M.D., M.R.C.P., F.R.C.Psych.

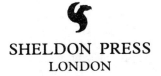

SHELDON PRESS
LONDON

First published in Great Britain in 1980 by
Sheldon Press, Marylebone Road, London NW1 4DU

Seventh impression 1991

Printed in England by Clays Ltd, St Ives plc

ISBN 0 85969 284 1

Contents

Introduction

When we talk to our friends, pick up a newspaper, listen to the radio or watch television we are bound to hear or see stress mentioned over and over again. Perhaps we hear it so often that it ceases to have any impact. A visitor from another planet coming across the word for the first time would have great difficulty in knowing what stress was, where it comes from and goes to, and how it is caused. From birth to death man seems to be surrounded by stress. A mother gets moody and depressed after childbirth; the stress of a difficult birth is blamed. The baby frequently cries and keeps the family awake at night. The father loses his temper and batters the child. Later, in court, the stress of coping with the new baby is blamed. He gets upset by the court appearance, gets headaches and feelings of tension and has a great deal of time off work. Stress is blamed again. Meanwhile his mother is convicted for shoplifting. She has never done this before and her defence is that the stress of the 'change of life' had made her act completely out of character. Soon after this her husband dies. He had only just been retired by his firm and his early death is blamed on the stress of being 'put on the scrapheap' before his time. His death provokes repercussions in his family and his wife becomes depressed because she cannot accept that he has gone. And so the round of stress goes on like a macabre dance. To cap it all, our planetary visitor will learn that as we now live in a 'stressful society' there is no way we can escape from the effect of stress.

He could draw several conclusions from his inquiry. First, stress is everywhere and, as it seems to be a recent phenomenon, it is probably a mysterious virus or bacterium that infects us from birth. Secondly, stress is unpleasant, and apparently has little to do with happy events. Thirdly, stress is somehow related to change. If he was a cynical observer he might reject all these conclusions and decide stress did not really exist but was merely a scapegoat. When anything went wrong in the lives of these strange humans the magical word stress was invoked as the universal excuse. Our visitor would also be surprised at the way in which we go about coping with and preventing stress. City businessmen who become stressed by sitting in offices making executive decisions all day are offered the opportunity of healthy outdoor exercise in the country, yet at the same time young people who spend all their working time in apparently healthy outdoor occupations are encouraged to continue further education so that they can better themselves. If they are 'successful' they may eventually reach a position where they can sit in offices all day making executive decisions and getting stressed, one of the perks of the job being the enjoyment of healthy exercise in the country at regular intervals! While trying to solve this curious paradox our visitor will be puzzled further by the tremendous differences in people's ideas of stress. Some will never take a journey by aeroplane because they find even the thought of flying too stressful to contemplate, while others take up hang-gliding as a hobby, considering it pleasant and exciting to fly through the air on an unpredictable course decided by the elements. Some are so concerned about motorized transport that they will not cross a busy street, a decision our visitor will probably regard as sensible after seeing traffic on our roads. Yet he will find a sport which depends on forcing these smelly, dangerous vehicles to the limits of speed and endurance round sharp bends which increase the risk of damage to man and car, and what is more, people pay to watch it because they find it pleasurable.

After our visitor has rubbed his eyes and scratched his

head in disbelief at the illogical behaviour of these stress-ridden Earthmen he might hope to be enlightened by looking at medical ways of treating stress. By now he will be quite certain that stress is a disease, for no healthy condition could cause people to behave in this way. At least he will find some consistency in this area but it is difficult to relate to the ideas about stress that he has come across earlier. Stress is reduced by techniques that are slowing-down rather than speeding-up. The slowing-down can be achieved in many ways, talking to people, taking pills, learning to relax, doing special exercises as in yoga and meditation, having a holiday or just taking it easy for a few days. As much of man's behaviour is geared to speeding-up rather than slowing-down, our visitor might be surprised, but by now he will probably have become used to the inconsistencies of this strange species. After surveying the range of treatments available for stress he could hardly be impressed by them. After all, if they worked why would everyone still be complaining about stress and its effects. His scepticism would be increased by looking at the large number of books and papers written about stress and its 'correct' treatment. After returning to his spaceship there would be only one way of describing what he had heard and seen without being accused of making it all up. The population of planet Earth are masochists. They make their lives unpleasant and then complain about it. They really enjoy this discomfort because all their efforts are designed to make it worse. They call this unpleasantness 'stress' because they are afraid to admit that they alone are the culprits.

Before you dismiss this conclusion as fanciful – read on. This book has been published as part of the 'Overcoming Common Problems' series but overcoming stress is not a realistic aim; although many set out to achieve it. In any case, stress has its good points as well as its bad ones and life without stress is not life, but death. Stress is not something outside us for which we can blame others. It comes from inside, and although we can often point to people, events and places as having a part to play in our reactions, they are not the only causes. We do not have to be the prisoners of our surroundings and to live with stress effectively we must either change our circumstances or ourselves. This is not an easy task and many of us find it easier to blame someone or something else which is beyond our control. Grumbling in this way will not help anyone, least of all you, and you will continue to suffer if you go on in this vein.

Even if you feel that there is nothing that can be done for your stress problems you may find something of value in this book. I do not promise any instant cures and you may be annoyed at some of the things I say along the way. But stay with me and think whether any of the advice I give might have a bearing on your own difficulties. I cannot give any personal prescriptions for coping with stress because, as you will see later, stress is a highly individual reaction. You have to make your decisions in the light of your own experience and situation. But I hope that after reading this book these decisions will be reached after careful thought and greater knowledge, and prove to work.

I

What is Stress?

The nonsense definition of stress goes something like this. 'Stress is feeling bad due to troubles beyond our control.' This includes the only two ideas about stress that are almost universal, that stress is unpleasant and that it is something that happens to us and which we can do little about. I want you to forget about these or any other preconceived ideas you may have about stress before we go any further, because they are only going to confuse you.

At this stage let us look at some examples of stress in action to see if there are any common features that will help us to find a satisfactory definition. All of them are described from real life, and it may help if we consider how we would feel if put through the same experiences.

A young man joins the Navy towards the end of the Second World War. He is sent out to the Far East and sees action in a battleship in the final year of the war against Japan. His job is to transfer ammunition from the hold to the guns above. The part of the hold where he works is open to the sky and he is surrounded by explosives. Above, Japanese kamikaze pilots try and weave their way through the barrage of anti-aircraft fire, looking for the chance to plunge to the decks in their human bombs to complete their suicide missions. The young man sees these planes and is reminded over and over again what will happen if a direct hit is scored on his ship. He cannot do anything to prevent it, and relies entirely on the accuracy of his fellow gunners. After six months of nerve-racking action he goes to pieces. He rarely sleeps but when he does he has nightmares of air attacks ending in a ball of flame when he wakes, sweating and terrified. He cannot concentrate and becomes inefficient at his job. He feels weak and has a series of symptoms, headaches, nausea, lack of appetite, loss of weight, nervous twitchings and blurring of vision. He is seen by a medical officer and sent back to England for shore duty.

Compare this stressful experience with one in another young man. He comes from a staid family who lay great emphasis on accuracy, reliability and security. The young man has no idea what to do when he leaves school but is persuaded by his parents to become a Civil Servant as this job requires all the qualities they hold most dear. In the absence of any alternative he reluctantly agrees and takes up a job as an assistant in a tax office, a job which has excellent prospects and is secure till retirement age. At first he works as a ledger clerk checking figures. The others in his office are older than him, but they are polite, well-spoken and helpful. He does his job well and is promoted to senior ledger clerk, now checking the figures of more important financial transactions. He continues to work with kind and considerate colleagues and his parents congratulate themselves on setting him forth on a worthwhile career. But after six months he is utterly bored with the apparent triviality of his job. He feels tyrannized by rows of meaningless figures, and irritated because they all have to balance on his ledger sheets. He gets curious impulses to upset the balance and falsify the figures, impulses to which he eventually succumbs. He sees his superior, hoping to be sacked, but instead is promoted. The pattern of boring, repetitive work among sympathetic, stolid people continues. At last he can stand it no longer. He gives up his job and goes to sea, and his parents are predictably horrified.

2

Finally, let us look at the case of a long-distance lorry driver who likes his job. It offers him variety and a degree of independence that he would not find elsewhere. True, at times he feels angry with other drivers on the road who seem not to appreciate the difficulties of driving a ten-ton lorry, but usually he enjoys sitting high above the road with so much throbbing power beneath him. He often prefers to drive for many hours at a stretch, although this means irregular meals and he knows it is frowned upon by the company. After several years of continual long-distance driving he starts to get pains in his stomach. They often wake him at night and trouble him during long drives. He finds milk drinks helpful and often takes them when he has the pain. But the pain gradually gets worse and he goes to see his doctor, who arranges for tests and referral to a specialist in hospital. The tests show that he has a duodenal ulcer. He discusses his future with the specialist and his own doctor and is advised to change his job as long-distance lorry driving is thought to be too stressful for him.

All three men have problems caused by stress but it is very difficult to find a common pattern in them. Most of us will sympathize strongly with the first man as he has been through a highly unpleasant experience which he has lost all power to control. Although most of us can tolerate the same degree of danger for short periods it becomes more difficult the longer it goes on, and sooner or later we all crack up. The second man will be more puzzling. Those of us who have tidy, methodical minds and prefer an organized routine in life will find it hard to understand why the young man should have reacted so strangely. Those who like more excitement in their lives and would not contemplate a career in the Civil Service will understand his reaction only too well and may be surprised he lasted as long as six months in the job. Our

3

third man will also provoke different feelings. Those of us who have never had serious indigestion or stomach pains will see him as a man with a satisfying job who just happens to develop a duodenal ulcer. Of course we may have read somewhere that duodenal ulcers are caused by stress but this will mean little to us unless we too have had indigestion when under stress. Then we would appreciate his symptoms only too well and probably have relieved them in similar ways.

The only common feature is conflict. This is shown mentally in the first two men and physically in the third. For some reason they and their surroundings do not mix properly and they cannot adapt in a healthy way. Beyond that they disagree. Many regard stress as something which puts us under increased pressure and forces us to act and think more quickly or intensely than we would like. But our man in his quiet office leisurely looking at figures is not under this kind of pressure. It is probably less than he would like. He finds it stressful because part of him shouts stridently through the conventional façade: 'Get me out of here, this isn't me!' This brings up one of the most important points about stress. Stress is not defined by what causes it but by a person's reaction to the cause, technically called the stressor. Those of us who cannot tolerate the Civil Service and have duodenal ulcers would probably find all three of the situations I described as stressful. By contrast, a healthy tax collector who likes his job and enjoys parachute jumping in his spare time (such people do exist) would find none of them stressful, although even he would find it difficult to remain settled in the battleship at war. This is why predicting stress is such a problem. It is easy to look back on an experience, knowing it has done harm, and to say it was the stress of X or Y that caused it. It is quite another matter to predict in advance that someone will be harmed by going through a particular experience. We may be right, but man has incredible powers of adaptation to the most unfavourable of settings.

A common fallacy about stress is that it is basically a nervous reaction. Our third example would not be included if this were true, because the first sign of stress that he experienced was the pain of his duodenal ulcer. Now if we had the key to his mind and could recall everything that he had been through over the years we would find that all was not as well as he made out, and his life-style was a stressful one. But the mind has a great ability to cast unwelcome feelings aside if they disagree with others that are strongly held. Our lorry driver could not be accused of dishonesty when he said he liked his job and found it satisfying. He was giving the truth according to his lights and showed no features suggesting a nervous reaction. But the mind and body are closely intertwined and stress can show itself in the body's reactions without the conscious mind being aware.

The best definition of stress I can give is that it is *the reaction of the mind and body to change*. This covers all the examples of stress that we have described and a great deal more. You will find other definitions of stress elsewhere and I do not pretend this is the only correct one. My definition is very broad and takes in a large range of reactions that many people do not find unpleasant even though they involve a great deal of change. The key issue is whether we adapt to the change when it takes place. If we do, the stress is hardly noticed; if we do not, the stress becomes distress. It persists and eventually breaks down mental and physical health. The definition includes all kinds of change, pleasant, unpleasant, exciting and boring. The stress of winning a fortune on the football pools can lead to distress in time if we do not adjust to it, and adjustment is often not as easy as we might think. If we do not adapt to the initial change, distress will go on continuously in the absence of further variation, but change always sets off the process. People react differently to change because they have different personalities and different ways of coping. Some situations are so unpleasant that the initial stress always moves on to distress. The situation of the young man on the battleship described earlier is so threatening that very few people could adapt to it completely, but that of working in a tax office involves only a slight change from normal in most people. Only a small number would find they cannot adapt to this and so become distressed. So when we say that something or other is stressful we really mean that the change it produces is large and most people would find difficulty in adjusting to it. We cannot say that *all* people without exception would become distressed. At the other end of the scale are changes which appear so small that we cannot see any possible problems in adapting, but they will appear much bigger changes to some people, and they cannot adjust easily. Each personality is different and we all have at least one weak spot, an Achilles' heel that can cause all sorts of problems.

We cannot alter people's basic personalities and so in living with stress we try and adjust as well as possible to all the changes going on about us. Many of these adjustments take place without our knowing much about them, but some bother us continually. The latter are the ones that make us feel 'under stress', force us to seek advice or take other forms of action to remove them. If we could always adjust to stress we should never become distressed. What makes some suffer from stress and others take it in their stride? Before answering this we need to know what goes on in our minds and bodies when we are under stress, and to decide when the stress is helpful and when it is harmful.

2

How Stress Affects your Mind and Body

Think of the time when you last had to run to catch a train or bus, or indeed took any vigorous exercise. You will have noticed a host of feelings which never concern you when you are relaxed.

Your breathing is deeper and quicker, and you cannot help being aware of your puffing and blowing. You are likely to be aware of your heart beating, something which you never notice normally. As well as feeling it hammering away in your chest you may also experience pulsating in your neck. Your muscles will be tense and active even if they are not involved in your athletic movements. This is best seen in your face, which is stretched into peculiar shapes by tension in its muscles, the agony of effort. If it is a hot day, you will sweat soon after the exercise begins. At first the sweating will be confined to your palms, soles, armpits and face, but as you get hotter beads of perspiration will spring up all over the surface of your body. On the other hand, your mouth will feel steadily drier the longer you are active, till at last your tongue will feel like coarse sandpaper in a hot kiln.

All these feelings are caused by your body trying to respond to the extra demands you are making, and yet at the same time compensating for these demands so that internal change is kept to a minimum. When you are active your muscles are working harder and need more oxygen from your blood. Automatic mechanisms (reflexes) come into play so that the heart pumps harder and quicker, and more of the blood is diverted to the muscles. If more blood goes to the muscles less has to go

7

elsewhere, and so the intestines and other digestive organs receive less. This is the main reason why your mouth feels dry when you are very active. The glands which keep the mouth moist with saliva are part of the digestive organs. When they receive less blood they get less active and your mouth is no longer well lubricated. Meanwhile your muscles work away and burn up most of the oxygen from your blood and replace it with carbon dioxide. When the level of carbon dioxide rises in the bloodstream your breathing is stimulated, so you puff and blow. This gets rid of the extra carbon dioxide and also takes more oxygen into the blood, which is pumped to the muscles. So each of the demands you set in motion by your energies is followed by your body but only at the cost of less activity elsewhere. You temporarily throw your body off balance by your dramatic changes but it quickly catches up. You will notice that it does not catch up completely as when you stop your exercise it takes a few minutes for your sweating to stop, your muscles to relax and your heart beat and breathing to return to normal. The fitter you are the shorter this time will be.

If you compare these feelings with those at a time when you felt emotionally keyed up in any way – angry, anxious, excited or frightened – you will recognize many similarities. You breathe more deeply and quickly, your heart pumps faster, you sweat on your face, palms and soles (but little elsewhere) and your muscles feel tense. The difference is that you are not usually physically energetic at this time. All these changes can go on without you moving from an armchair. They are all part of the preparation for action. Your body receives impulses from your mind saying 'I realize you are a bit slow on the up-take so I'm giving you ample warning that I'm liable to swing into emergency action in the very near future!' So the body primes its emergency systems and anticipates

8

action even if it never arrives. Physical and emotional stress are essentially the same, except that emotional stress seldom reaches the same intensity in its demands on the body. It is also worth remembering that the body does not take any notice of the kind of emotion being shown. It makes no difference whether you are red in the face from anger or hot and bothered with embarrassment, the body reacts in the same way.

These healthy reactions of the body to stress are mainly controlled by a special part of the nervous system, called the autonomic nervous system. Autonomic means self-governing, and the name illustrates that the system organizes itself without any interference from outside. There are two parts to the system which normally remain in balance. The sympathetic part is the one that gears you for action and makes you aware of your body function. It is sometimes called the 'fight and flight' system because most emergencies involve running away from a danger or advancing towards conflict. It can be brought into operation fairly quickly because in addition to nervous stimulation there are hormones secreted into the blood which rapidly pass round the body and stimulate the organs for action. The chief hormone is adrenalin, which stimulates the heart and muscles and makes you aware of its effects in only a few seconds.

By contrast there is the parasympathetic system. Its job is best summed up by the phrase 'rest and digest'. When you are most calm outwardly your parasympathetic system is at its most energetic. It is responsible for rest and sleep, for organizing the digestion and breakdown of food, storing up supplies in the body ready for use in an emergency, and for keeping everything ticking over nicely. It takes much longer to get into operation than the sympathetic system and works at its best when there is least interruption, usually when you are asleep.

9

If you think of a country at war and then compare it at peace you get a good analogy of the two different systems. The declaration of war is an emergency and mobilization is urgent. As quickly as possible factories have to be converted from the needs of peace to those of war. So production of cars, washing machines, refrigerators and farm machinery is cut down and replaced by tanks, guns, armoured cars and battleships. People are transferred from their jobs to the armed services and most of the country's budget goes into the war effort. In peace-time the priorities are different. People are concerned with getting a higher standard of living and making their lives more comfortable, so many more goods to achieve these ends are made for sale. Apart from the obvious differences in activity between the two systems you will probably have noticed another. The peace-time system is much more balanced than the wartime one. That is why you hear so much fuss about the balance of payments. If a country at peace cannot balance what it sells and buys from abroad it runs into trouble with its economy. A country on a war footing is different. It is almost expected to get out of balance, to run up debts which will be paid for after the war, which is why post-war credits, war bonds and other arrangements for paying for the war become necessary. The policy becomes 'let us put everything into the fight so we can win as quickly as possible', even if this means being in hock for years afterwards. When the war is over the balancing peace-time system has to pay off these debts as well as trying to satisfy the demand for improved living standards.

The sympathetic system puts the body temporarily out of balance when it comes into operation, and the parasympathetic system has to make up for it afterwards. The activity of the sympathetic system is part of healthy stress when it is only temporary and can soon be corrected. But if the sympathetic stimulation goes on for too long unopposed by the parasympathetic it becomes impossible to get compensation afterwards and the stress is no longer healthy.

The key difference between healthy and harmful stress is that in healthy stress there is rapid adjustment to the change and in harmful stress there is little or no adjustment. This point is critical to understanding and coping with stress. Remember our definition of stress – the reaction of mind and body to change. We are surrounded by changes but have no trouble in adjusting to most of them. It is only those changes that we have no answer to that lead to harmful stress, the sort of stress that people complain about and which causes physical and mental suffering. Let us see how uncompensated stress can do harm.

Remember the man with the duodenal ulcer that we came across in the last chapter. He was not consciously aware of his 'fight and flight' mechanisms coming into action while driving his lorry. This is because the stimulation of his sympathetic nervous system was only a mild one, but it persisted. When this happens the body has another trick up its sleeve. Another group of hormones, the main one being cortisone, is secreted into the blood and sets the body's defences at a higher level so it can withstand the stress. But this cannot go on indefinitely and sooner or later these defences fail. A well-known expert on stress, Dr Hans Selye, first described the three stages of the 'adaptation syndrome'. The first alarm stage is the initial sympathetic reaction for fight and flight. The second stage is that of resistance. The stress has been partly dealt with by the body but if it continues the resistance has to be kept up, throwing a strain on the body's defences. The third stage is exhaustion. The body, or part of it, gives up the fight and dies.

Which parts of the body are affected varies from person to person and also depends on the type of stress. It would be wrong to think of a duodenal ulcer just being caused by the stress of driving a lorry for long distances. Two other stresses are the irregular hours of work, for if you work for sixteen hours a day your parasympathetic system does not get enough time to do its work, and irregular meals, often of the wrong sort of food. A combination of the three stresses picks out the duodenum, the part of the intestine just below the stomach, as the weakest link in the body's chain of defences. The cells on its surface die and the acid from the stomach juices burns a hole in the lining. For the ulcer to heal the parasympathetic nervous system needs plenty of time to get the stomach and intestine back into balance, so a combination of regular meals with bland foods, change to a more settled job and greater relaxation are needed. Of course the ulcer can also be helped by taking medicines or having surgery but is likely to recur if other adjustments in life are not made as well.

Emotional stress may not be involved at all. For example, the physical stress of being overweight can cause a great deal of damage on its own. If you are ten stones overweight your bones and your joints have to work much harder in supporting and transporting the extra load, a load which they are not equipped to cope with indefinitely. After resisting valiantly for years the linings of your joints wear out. The roughened surfaces rub together and produce the pain and swelling of arthritis. If you told an overweight person with arthritis that he was suffering from stress he would probably be highly indignant. Fat people are usually placid, and as stress implies 'nerves' he would deny any connection. But stress is stress whatever its source and the body makes no allowances.

This does not mean that all bodily disease is due to or provoked by stress. Many conditions such as diabetes pass down from one generation to another and there is very little we can do to prevent them. But some diseases which apparently come out of the blue are caused by stress which you have ignored, dismissed or denied. I hope you will have a good idea whether you are ignoring stress at your peril by the time you finish this book. But this does not mean that all unexplained disease is caused by stress. There is still much to learn about the causes of many diseases and because stress is all around us we are sometimes tempted into blaming it for illnesses that we cannot understand. It is also difficult to decide which type of stress is most important in a disease. Take high blood pressure. We have already found out that the sympathetic nervous system stimulates the heart and circulation and in emotional and physical stress the extra work may put the heart into failure. But high blood pressure is also caused by our arteries becoming clogged and inflexible so the heart has to work harder to pump blood round the body. The clogging up of arteries is made worse by eating too much fat in your diet, being overweight or smoking cigarettes, all of which are physical stresses. In trying to counteract the stress we can ask the patient to take life easier so that his sympathetic system receives less stimulation, but we run the danger of reducing his activity so much that he sits all day doing nothing apart from eating, puts on weight and clogs his arteries still further. If on the other hand we ask him to take some healthy exercise in the form of jogging, we run the risk of putting extra pressure on his already overworked heart. So we can make one form of stress worse by making another better, and simple slogans such as 'jogging is good for your health' cannot apply to everybody.

Cancer has sometimes been linked to stress but clear

evidence of a relationship does not exist. In cancer, cells in the body do not die but grow without any control until they destroy other cells. Although stress can lead to the death of cells we have no direct evidence that they stimulate their uncontrolled growth. The cause of only a few types of cancer is known and we cannot put the rest down to stress. Nevertheless there are some dramatic instances in which inoperable cancer has apparently been cured without any explanation. It is too early to tell whether stress has any part to play in this.

Stress can also cause symptoms that fool us into thinking we have physical disease when we are really quite well. Our sympathetic nervous systems stimulate our bodies and produce feelings that are very similar to those of real disease. The irritating awareness of the heart beating (and missing beats), difficulty in breathing, nausea and sickness, tension in arms and legs, headache and giddiness, interfere with our thoughts and actions. We often feel anxious and upset at these times. It annoys us because there is often no reason to feel anxious. Sometimes only one or two of these bodily feelings bother us and most of our anxiety is about these symptoms. When this happens it is very easy to get the idea that you have a physical illness. Your body is behaving in a way which is unfamiliar and you do not feel well. This is alarming and you make an appointment with your doctor to have a 'full physical check-up'. (It is interesting that people with other health problems seldom ask for this; they just present their symptoms.) Now this may seem a perfectly reasonable thing to do but in most cases the outcome of the consultation is far from satisfactory. The doctor examines you and finds no evidence of physical illness. He tells you so. At one level you are pleased but at another you are suspicious. If you have no physical disease then what is the cause of these nasty feelings? You blurt out the question, 'you don't think I'm imagining this, doctor?' You don't want to appear to be wasting his time and yet you want more than simple reassurance. You may even feel angry or suspect the doctor of incompetence.

In fact your doctor is in a difficult position. He cannot be absolutely sure that you have no physical disease but he knows from the pattern of your symptoms that they are much more likely to be due to stress. This does not mean the symptoms are imaginary. They are real to you and there are genuine changes going on in the body which cause them, but they are not the changes of physical disease, at least not at this stage. If your doctor is not sure about this, and particularly if you go back to him repeatedly with the same complaint, he may refer you to a specialist of a hospital. The specialist has the advantages of a fuller range of tests as well as having expert knowledge. So if, for example, you have palpitations you are likely to be referred to a heart specialist. He carries out all the tests necessary to make sure you have no heart disease and again reassures you. But often this reassurance is no more satisfying than the reassurance you got from your own doctor, unless of course by this time your symptoms have gone away. The danger is that you will get started on a round of medical (and non-medical) consultations hoping that one of them will find your undiscovered disease. If you persevere long enough (and spend enough money) you may finally get the 'disease' named. But it is not a real disease and the name may just be a description of your main problem in Latin and Greek, a name which sounds impressive but says very little.

If your doctor recognizes that these feelings are related to psychological stresses he may still have some difficulty in talking about them to you. The mere mention of the word 'psychological' implies to some people that they do imagine symptoms and that they are 'neurotic'. So however the interview goes it is likely that you will be far from satisfied with your visit. If you get upset and angry your symptoms will trouble you still more and you may feel worse after the interview than you did before.

Doctors call these complaints psychosomatic or 'functional' disorders. They prefer not to deal with them because there is a limited amount that specialized medical knowledge can do for them, and everyone prefers satisfied to dissatisfied customers. Later we shall discuss ways in which you can go about assessing and treating these problems but at this stage I want you to appreciate that although these troubles may appear to be easily treated they are really quite difficult.

Do these bodily feelings cause real disease if they go on for long enough? This is the question that naturally follows from what we have said earlier about stress, but curiously, the answer seems to be no. People can go on for years worrying about their hearts skipping beats, pumping like steam-hammers, and making the chest feel sore without real heart disease developing, and the same applies to the other kinds of symptom. Some doctors feel it might even be of value to have these symptoms, because they warn you when you are doing too much and make sure you pace yourself in all your activities. So although it may seem strange, the people who are often most worried about their bodies are the ones who should have the least cause for concern. Having said that, we cannot regard these feelings as healthy. They cause worry and annoyance and we would love to be rid of them. But most of the ill-health is to the mind and not to the organs in the body. I am not just putting the usual doctor's line of reassurance here. There is no connection between these bodily feelings of stress and physical disease.

Stress can be involved in the cause of physical disease and the first evidence of disease is a bodily symptom. It may be the pain of a duodenal ulcer, the headache and sickness of migraine or the difficulty in breathing of the asthmatic. Emotional stress alone does not cause any of these diseases; they are due to a combination of factors. But emotional stress alone is the most frequent cause of psychosomatic complaints.

Once a disease has developed, emotional factors can make it worse, and the diseases that are most affected are ones which affect the parts of the body most involved by the stimulation of the sympathetic nervous system. So it is advisable for people with heart disease to avoid all types of emotional stress because it makes extra demands on the heart, but no such advice needs to be given in anaemia as it is not affected by the emotions. Asthma, bowel and skin disease, high blood pressure, peptic ulcer and migraine are all sensitive to emotional pressures and relapses can be caused by them. It is much easier to make changes in the diet, to take tablets, or to move to a new part of the country than it is to cut down on stress, but it can be done.

The focus of stress is often the mind rather than the body. Again there are many ways in which stress can show itself. It is particularly difficult to adjust to severe changes if they catch us unprepared.

If a close relative dies suddenly we are faced with immediate and severe stress. We are forced to adjust to a change which we might never have contemplated. Adjustment is painful and hard but usually we adapt in the end. But sometimes if the task seems too much we take the easy way out. Although at one level we accept the loss, at an emotional level we pretend it has not happened. The distress and unhappiness that we should be feeling is not shown at all. Everyone says how well we are taking the loss because we do not give an embarrassing public display of emotion, and the stiff upper lip appears to have won again. But it has not. Underneath the calm exterior the distressing emotions are rumbling like a volcano ready to erupt, and doing much greater damage than if they had been allowed expression. Many months later the volcano does indeed erupt, in the form of mental illness. Severe depression is the most common illness after loss but it is quite different from ordinary sadness. Feelings of terrible guilt and unworthiness torment the victim, the future looks absolutely hopeless, and death by suicide is felt to be the only solution. Silent stress has done its damage. The problem is now much worse than if the stress had been shown openly. We could not have a better example of the benefits of stress than the strong expressions of sorrow, desperation and tears that are normal in grief. They are very stressful in the short-term but by opening the dam of the emotions all the blockages to long-term adjustment are washed away in the spate. When calm returns we can build up a new life again, while still accepting the fact of the loss.

An even better but much less common example of the mind 'shutting off' when it has to cope with something it considers too unpleasant is the condition which used to be called shell-shock. It is hard to conceive of something more stressful to the mind than fighting in the trenches during the First World War. Soldiers lived for months in intolerable conditions under constant threat of death. The terrible cry 'over the top' when they had to advance out of the safety of the trenches and run towards the enemy meant death to many and those who lived only exchanged one set of squalid conditions for another. Small wonder that the natural reaction was to go backwards rather than forwards. Duty and instinct were in conflict, and at times instinct won. The mind cried:

'Enough is enough. I can no longer tolerate the stress you are putting me under and am going to take independent action to reduce it.' So the affected soldier went into a state in which he forgot who and where he was or what he was doing, and walked instinctively backwards from the trenches in a daze. His conscious mind was not involved in this but the military authorities would be unlikely to believe this when he was 'captured' and put on trial for desertion.

Although we seldom come across such severe stress in peace-time there are times when our minds can react in the same sort of way. Many people do not remember everything about a serious accident, a fire or a similar episode even though they are conscious all the time. The sight of bodies being crushed or burnt, and the cries of agony and distress, are too much for our senses to bear. So at the time we shut them off from consciousness. But these sights and sounds still leave an impression and we have to adjust to them in time. Occasionally we get into trouble for not accepting what our senses tell us and acting at once. When people are said to be paralysed with fear they are often not frightened at all, but so overwhelmed by stresses that they do nothing. Like an electrical instrument put on overload, they 'blow a fuse' and wait. This can have disastrous consequences. It has been suspected that lives are lost unnecessarily when aeroplanes crash-land and catch fire. Even when there is time for all the passengers to escape through the emergency chutes some stay glued to their seats with their safety belts securely fixed. They cannot adjust quickly enough to the change from being relaxed and secure to an emergency in which their lives can be saved only by their own reactions. The transfer of complete faith in the air crew back to personal responsibility takes place too quickly, and whilst they may respond to instructions from others they are incapable of thinking for themselves. It is only helpful to be calm in the face of danger if we fully realize what the danger is and how we are going to deal with it.

The most common mental component of harmful stress is abnormal anxiety. Short lasting feelings of anxiety are often helpful even though they may seem unpleasant at the time. The student working for an exam is likely to work harder if he is anxious about doing well. The journalist who is made anxious because he has to write a story in time for the next edition of his paper is likely to work all the faster. The mother who gets anxious about her son playing in the road will move him to a safer place and so reduce the risk of an accident. The list is endless; without anxiety all our lives would be the poorer. But in harmful stress anxiety is so crippling it stops us from doing anything constructive.

The student who gets an abnormal fear of examinations (a phobia) gets so anxious about the test that he goes to pieces. He looks at the question paper and finds the words have no meaning. He cannot remember all the work he has spent weeks revising. When he raises his pen to write his hand shakes so much every word is illegible. A little anxiety is good for us but too much is deadly. Once it gets out of hand it seems to be with us constantly. Instead of being turned on by demand it surrounds us like a cloud. When this happens we cannot say what we are anxious about and make feeble excuses to satisfy others. But in reality every little change is taken as a serious threat. The sudden noise of a bell ringing, a knock on the door, an innocent item on the television, a telephone call, are all full of hidden dangers and create still more anxiety. It is as though we are stumbling through a dark tunnel, not knowing where we are going and what horrors lie ahead, so every signal, no matter how small, is filled with foreboding.

If anxiety continues at this pitch for any length of time we become inefficient shadows of our normal selves. Unfortunately we respond in exactly the same way to night-time anxiety, which shows as insomnia. We cannot get to sleep until the anxieties of the day have subsided, and it can take many hours for this to happen if you have been strung up all day. Lack of sleep results, so concentration and efficiency are lost the next day and add to the effects of anxiety. We also become irritable and often quite different from our normal personalities. We snap and snarl, find fault with everyone except ourselves, and start petty arguments which waste even more time. Although we get angry with ourselves for behaving in this kind of way we do not seem to be able to prevent it. Because we are not coping we can easily get down-hearted and depressed. We feel sorry for ourselves, feel like crying, think the future seems hopeless and lose all energy. This makes us cope even less well than before. So instead of adjusting to the change we make it worse. Technically this is called positive feedback. 'Feedback' is a term we shall come across later and we need to be quite clear what it means. When something changes in a system, feedback can make the change less (negative feedback) or more (positive feedback). Most healthy stress involves negative feedback and only lasts a short time. Anxiety which gets out of control involves positive feedback. The problem is like a snowball rolling down a hill. To begin with it is small and manageable but as it rolls it gets larger, picking up more and more snow, and as it gets heavier it gets out of control. All the compensatory techniques of normal stress fail and you finish up by breaking down. A nervous breakdown is not really a medical term but it aptly describes the state we get into. The normal mechanisms of our mental function pack up and everything stops. Even though the breakdown may seem to have no purpose it at least stops us from doing more damage to ourselves, and is often the signpost to recovery. But because it happens when everything is out of control we often do things that are completely out of character. Many people seem to realize at one level of their minds that something must be done to stop themselves rushing headlong from crisis to crisis and bring the final act of breakdown on themselves. The upright housewife who has always been the best of citizens takes goods from a shop without paying for them, the quiet respectable worker who normally gives in to authority fetches his employer a punch in the ribs, the proper young lady who is a stickler for etiquette takes an overdose of pills and finishes up with the indignity of the stomach pump. It seems as though the only way we can put a stop to this self-generating stress is by doing something which is quite the opposite of our normal behaviour. And it works. Although the immediate consequences of a breakdown are unpleasant they allow us to look at our problem in a different light, to see things that we were blind to before, to realize that blaming outside influences for our troubles was wrong, as we alone were responsible. For the first time for many weeks we can think clearly because the pressure has been taken away.

Most of the harmful stress we come across in life is of this type. We ask too much of ourselves when we are under pressure. Our bodies and minds cannot keep up with the speed and intensity of the demands we make upon them. But it would be wrong to assume that stress only results from too much pressure. Equally severe stress can result from too little stimulation. You might find this hard to believe but this is because you have probably never been severely under-stimulated. When people have been placed in situations of this kind they react in a most surprising way. Imagine being suspended in a tank of warm water with your head covered and a breathing mask over your face, or even being confined to bed in a sound-proofed room. This may sound a blissful way of whiling away the hours but it turns out not to be. Very few people can tolerate these conditions for more than two or three days because they are so unpleasant. After a few hours they have difficulty in concentrating, and their minds wander from one subject to another. Odd ideas, or fantasies, flit across the mind, and if you happen to be suspended in water they are frequently sexual in nature. Time gets out of joint, minutes seem like hours, and when they cannot tolerate the conditions any longer people are amazed to find that they have only been confined for a few days, not weeks or months. Instead of feeling relaxed subjects often feel tense and have headaches and other pains. They feel nervous and sometimes become terrified and panic-stricken. This is hardly surprising when the shape or weight of your body seems to be changing, when you develop the belief that your mind is being controlled by people outside or that you are being deliberately punished. These feelings are the most serious effects of prolonged isolation and take some time to disappear even when the isolation is over.

None of us would find these feelings pleasant and it is not surprising that volunteers who think they could do with a long rest (and get paid for it into the bargain) ask to come out of isolation long before they originally intended. When they are back in the land of normal living again they talk about their experiences as though they had been through the severe stress of armed battle. Although this may at first seem odd, when we consider our definition of stress it is entirely predictable. Stress, you will remember, is the reaction of the mind and body to change, and change can be less or more. Even the proverbial man who goes on banging his head against a brick wall experiences a minor form of stress when he stops using his head as a hammer although it is much less than if he continues. Most change which leads to less stimulation than previously is mildly pleasurable, but if the difference is great and if under-stimulation is prolonged, the mind and body react in just the same stressful way as when they are over-stimulated. Although it is not every day you are likely to have the opportunity of being suspended in warm water with only a breathing tube for company or even lying in a sound-proofed room, you will probably have experienced situations in real life that are similar if not so extreme. Boredom is often the first sign of under-stimulation, and who can claim that he or she has never been bored? If you are bored and relaxed you can escape further boredom by dropping off to sleep, but if you already have had more than enough sleep it is another matter. Often when convalescing from an illness we go through a stage when we feel fit but are still confined to bed. We are fed up with reading, writing letters or doing crosswords and we can think of nothing that we would like more than to stretch our legs and take a walk in the open air. This is the stage of illness we often find most frustrating, and during which we are the most difficult of patients. We are irritable and snappy, complain of tension, aches and pains, and show all the signs of harmful stress.

The same stressful effects are shown whenever we are forced to go on doing the same thing for week after week without any prospect of change. This is the curious paradox of stress. Although it is the reaction to change it can also be reaction to lack of change. This is because a life which repeats itself in the same way as the hands of a clock retrace each minute and hour of the day becomes a life of boredom and under-stimulation. Every movement and act is predictable and eventually becomes automatic.

A life of novelty becomes one of boredom and the harmful stress cycle is set in motion.

Unfortunately far too many of us think we are compelled to go through life without much change. We do things that we would prefer not to do and after a little while cannot see any alternative. There are ways of escaping the deadlock of boredom and we shall discuss these later. But at this stage we need to be reminded that although the highly pressured business executive tends to come to mind whenever we think of stress, exactly the same degree of stress can be experienced by the bored housewife, spending her day cleaning, shopping, and preparing meals in a continuous round of duty. If she would choose to do none of these things if she had alternatives, and if her family take her for granted so that she never gets any respite, she and her executive equivalent will both be paying visits to the doctor for their stress disease to be treated.

Each of us has a level of stress with which we are most happy, one which satisfies our need for novelty yet allows us to make adjustments to change smoothly and completely. Because we differ from each other we should not allow others to decide this level for us. We are not pre-packaged machines set to operate at the flick of a switch, although the speeches of politicians, the slogans of advertising and the techniques of mass communication sometimes assume we are. The pressures on us to conform have always been great in human society but now it is not so much the heavy hand of the dictator as soft talking through the television screen that is the main threat to our independence. If we give in to these pressures about half of us will find that the stresses which we come across are at or near our optimum level, but the other half will find they are either too low or too high. To decide whether the stress in your life is healthy or harmful there is no alternative to using yourself as the yardstick. By all means listen to what others have to say but remember that you are the only one that feels the symptoms of stress and are in the best position to judge whether they are doing harm.

How do you decide your ideal level of stress? No, it is not a question of trial and error. Your personality is the key. Personality is not a showbiz term pretending to tell you whether or not you have star quality, but a word describing the sort of person you are. Now you may have very clear ideas of the sort of person you are. Alternatively, you may think of personality as a meaningless term thought up by psychologists. Whatever your views, read the next chapter with an open mind, and prepare to be surprised.

3

Stress and Personality

When we are asked to describe someone's personality we often find it difficult. The questioner is asking what kind of person is X or Y, and while it is easy to describe their physical appearance it is difficult to put personality into words. We often finish up using bland words like nice, pleasant, all right, and okay, which mean virtually nothing. Yet we all have a mental image of someone's personality, the particular combination of features that is as unique as a fingerprint and much more interesting. While everyone is different, there are some features that tend to go together and form types of personality.

If you would like to find out your type of personality you should answer the questionnaire which follows. For each item you are given seven possible replies (indicated by the letters *a–g*). Decide which of the seven comes closest to describing your reaction and note this as your *first* choice. Do the same again after deciding your *second* and *third* choice. Try and take your past experience as well as your present feelings into account before making your answer. Please answer as honestly as possible; there are no right or wrong replies. Even if none of the replies fits your particular reaction pick the three which are most close.

1. You are in a hurry and about to cross a busy road in a large town. Do you:

    (*a*) feel angry with drivers if you are kept waiting?

(b) only cross when the way is quite clear, no matter how long you have to wait?

(c) only cross when other people are crossing?

(d) rush across, dodging the traffic?

(e) only cross when traffic has stopped moving as drivers can never be trusted?

(f) try to get the traffic to stop, making it clear you are in a hurry?

(g) look for a zebra crossing and cross by one even if it means a detour?

2. You are offered alcoholic drinks at a party where most of the guests are strangers to you. Do you:

(a) accept one drink but rarely accept a second?

(b) accept the drink that most of the others are drinking?

(c) drink till you feel calm and more confident?

(d) drink as much as you can get?

(e) refuse the drink unless you know exactly what is in it?

(f) drink till you feel happy?

(g) refuse the offer?

3. You have a choice of jobs, each of similar pay. Which of the following would you consider important in making your choice?

(a) good prospects of promotion.

(b) easy work which makes few demands on you.

(c) security.

(d) good holidays.

(e) working alone.

(f) working with people who understand you.

(g) a set routine.

4. You are waiting in a queue and there is no immediate prospect of the queue moving. Do you:

   (a) keep looking at your watch and get impatient?

   (b) just relax while waiting?

   (c) worry about one thing or another?

   (d) prefer not to wait and do something else instead?

   (e) look at other people in the queue?

   (f) talk to other people in the queue?

   (g) work out problems in your mind while waiting?

5. You have just been told that you have won first prize in a lottery. What is your immediate reaction?

   (a) to work out how you will spend your winnings.

   (b) to continue what you were doing as though nothing had happened.

   (c) to take something to calm you down.

   (d) to have a party to celebrate.

   (e) to worry about possible publicity.

   (f) to tell a close friend or relative.

   (g) to check the number of the lottery ticket.

6. You have just been interviewed for a new job and told you were unsuccessful. Do you:

   (a) feel angry because they did not appreciate your true worth?

(b)   forget about it immediately?

(c)   feel tense and miserable?

(d)   go and have a drink to forget about it?

(e)   feel the interviewer had a grudge against you?

(f)   get it off your chest by talking to somebody about it?

(g)   go over the interview in your mind to see where you went wrong?

7.   You have just had an argument with a friend and are not on speaking terms. Do you:

(a)   forget about it by concentrating hard on something else?

(b)   take it in your stride and ignore it?

(c)   find it difficult to stop yourself shaking?

(d)   feel like hitting somebody?

(e)   wonder why people seem to turn against you?

(f)   tell someone else what happened?

(g)   go over the argument again and again in your mind?

8.   You are planning a holiday. Do you:

(a)   go somewhere new which presents a challenge?

(b)   go where you can rest and relax?

(c)   go somewhere which is safe and secure?

(d)   make no plans and hope for the best?

(e)   prefer to go where you can be on your own?

(f)   decide where you are going but leave the details to someone else?

(g) prefer to plan in detail so that every day is accounted for?

9. A close member of your family has failed to arrive home at the expected time. Do you:

(a) use the opportunity to catch up on some work?

(b) feel unconcerned?

(c) get very worried indeed?

(d) only realize he or she is late after they arrive home?

(e) feel suspicious about the reasons for the delay?

(f) feel all right as long as there is someone else to talk to?

(g) work out in your mind all the possible causes for the delay?

10. You are about to buy some new clothes. Do you choose:

(a) the best clothes, even if they are the most expensive?

(b) clothes which are the most comfortable?

(c) clothes which are in your nearest shop, even if they are not ideal?

(d) the first clothes which take your fancy?

(e) clothes which are such that you do not stand out in a crowd?

(f) the latest fashion?

(g) clothes which are very similar to your present ones?

11. You have just been informed that a close friend of yours has been injured in an accident. What is your reaction?

(a) to get details of the accident and organize help.

(b) to reassure others as much as possible.

(c) to feel very upset.

(d) to feel glad that it was not you.

(e) to find out who was to blame.

(f) to visit him (or her) as soon as possible.

(g) to work out in your mind how it could have been avoided.

12. You have just been introduced to a stranger whom you will be working with closely in the future. What sort of person would you like them to be?

(a) someone with ambition, energy and drive.

(b) someone who is easy-going and placid.

(c) someone who makes you feel at ease.

(d) someone who is lively and exciting.

(e) someone you can trust.

(f) someone who is interesting to talk to.

(g) someone who is reliable and conscientious.

13. You are working and have just been presented with an unusual problem. Do you:

(a) have to get it sorted out before you can return to your normal work?

(b) deal with it in exactly the same way as your ordinary work?

(c) find it upsets your concentration?

(d) prefer dealing with it instead of doing your ordinary work?

(e) make certain it is your responsibility before dealing with it?

(*f*)   usually ask advice before dealing with it?

(*g*)   only deal with it when you have completely finished the work you are doing?

14.   You have nearly finished work for the day and have a severe headache. Do you:

(*a*)   take an aspirin and keep on working until the job is done no matter how bad your headache is?

(*b*)   stop working and rest till the headache goes away?

(*c*)   take an aspirin and something to calm your nerves?

(*d*)   have an alcoholic drink?

(*e*)   think you have been made to work too hard?

(*f*)   take an aspirin immediately and lie down until it takes effect?

(*g*)   stop work temporarily but continue as soon as the headache is better?

15.   You are listening to somebody who takes a long time to explain things. Do you:

(*a*)   try and work out what he means and interrupt him by repeating your interpretation so that you save time?

(*b*)   wait till he has finished no matter how long he (or she) takes?

(*c*)   worry when you will be allowed to speak?

(*d*)   interrupt and talk about something completely different?

(*e*)   wonder if he (or she) is making fun of you?

(*f*)   stop listening but pretend to be still listening?

(*g*)   listen carefully to everything that is said and reorganize it in your mind?

Now add up the total scores for each separate letter throughout the questionnaire. For each first choice score three points, for each second choice score two points, and for each third choice score one point. The letter with the highest number of points indicates your personality type. The types and their matching letters are:

(a) ambitious type   (e) suspicious type

(b) placid type   (f) dependent type

(c) worrying type   (g) fussy type.

(d) carefree type

You may get equal scores for two personality types, in which case you should add up the total of first choices for each of them, choosing the one that has the most.

All these personality types have unattractive as well as pleasant features, but I would like you to stay with the type that the questionnaire has decided for you, even if you feel it is not an accurate one. You never know, you might learn something new about yourself as we proceed.

Let us take a closer look at each of these personalities. I am going to describe some typical examples of each one, the kind of people who would score over 30 points for the appropriate personality in the questionnaire. To match with the letters from the questionnaire they are named after the first seven letters of the Greek alphabet.

THE AMBITIOUS TYPE

Mr Alpha has done well in life. He has always been an active and energetic man. He cannot stand being still for more than a few minutes and when he is not working he is always busy with one activity or another. He is con-

34

scientious and has very high standards, and often gets annoyed with others for not coming up to his expectations. Time is a problem in his life; he never seems to have enough. At work he is always rushing from one appointment to another and has no time to relax. He gets impatient easily, talks quickly and aggressively and tends to frighten people. He is dominant in his relationships and likes to control those around him. Because he has worked so hard and had so much energy he is now the managing director of his company, which has become a much larger concern since he took over. People are proud of what he has done but wish he would take things more easily now.

THE PLACID TYPE

Mr Beta is a quiet man, and many people say he is lazy. Although he did well at school he did not like the idea of further education with more examinations and took a job as a farm labourer. He is now a market gardener and has a reasonable standard of living but his wife keeps telling him how much better off they would be if only he worked harder. Often in the summer when he should be busy in the garden he says the weather is too good for work and goes off to the seaside with his family. His favourite hobby is fishing and he spends hours at a canal near his home even though he never catches anything of importance. He is bad with money and his wife has to keep the accounts or bills are not paid. He never seems to worry about anything and seldom gets involved in arguments, and because of this some people find him boring. Although he has always been good at sport he has never won any competitions and cannot see the point of them. He says he does things because he enjoys doing them and for no other reason.

THE WORRYING TYPE

Miss Gamma has always been 'highly strung'. She has little self-confidence and from an early age has been worried about doing things wrong. Even when everything is going well she is worried about the future and consequently finds it difficult to relax. She likes to organize her life so she can avoid being faced with new problems which only make her nervous, but as life is not predictable and as she is not a very good organizer she usually finds whenever there is a crisis or unexpected hitch in her life she gets very panicky and sometimes feels as if she will go to pieces. She works as a secretary and although she is a good one she always worries that she may let people down. She used to think that she would feel more confident once she was in control of her job but it never seems to happen. Although she is capable of getting a better job she is worried about the strain of increased responsibility and prefers to stay in her present position. She has been engaged to be married for a year. Her boyfriend is very understanding but at times they have had serious disagreements, chiefly about sex. She is afraid that she might be frigid and has avoided sexual relations because of her doubts and fears, although she pretends to her boyfriend that her decision is a moral one. At times she wonders whether she can cope with marriage and also doubts her ability to look after children. Whenever she looks into the future there appear to be more anxieties crowding in on her.

THE CAREFREE TYPE

Mr Delta is a disc jockey at a local radio station, but he has also worked as a van-driver, racing mechanic and salesman. His favourite saying is 'variety is the spice of life' and he acts on this by moving round the country from one job to another. His friends keep advising him to think about the future and settle down but he cannot understand their concern. He enjoys life now and does not see why the future should be any different. In his spare time he likes parachute jumping and particularly relishes the feeling of flying unsupported through the air in the short time between jumping from the aeroplane and pulling the rip-cord of his parachute. He had hoped to go into rally driving when he was a mechanic but had so many driving accidents that no insurance company would cover him. He liked the excitement and novelty of his job as a disc jockey at first but now is beginning to find this a little tedious and already is thinking of another change. He drinks more alcohol than most people and is sometimes violent when he has had too much. He has had many girlfriends in the past but usually ends each relationship after a few months. Several years ago one of his girlfriends became pregnant and he arranged an illegal abortion. He tells all his girlfriends that he has no intention of getting married but they still get closely involved. The thought of living with one person for the rest of his life makes him shudder.

THE SUSPICIOUS TYPE

Mr Epsilon is a schoolteacher. He is dedicated to his job and takes it very seriously, and feels more at home with children than does with adults. Since his early years he has been concerned what people think of him and cannot help thinking that they criticize him behind his back. He distrusts most people and is careful not to reveal his true feelings until he knows someone really well. When he is criticized he takes it very badly and thinks about it for weeks afterwards. Even when he is not being criticized he finds double meanings in things that are said to him and always takes the least favourable interpretation. His wife has to be careful what she says to him because he bears a grudge easily and if annoyed he often refuses to talk to her for days on end. Whenever he has moved house or changed to a new school it has taken many months for him to settle down, and he goes through a phase when he is even more prickly and sensitive than usual. If he is asked to take on different duties at school he thinks he is being criticized for being incompetent and becomes moody. But at home with his family he is usually settled and relaxed, and is happiest when playing with his children. He trusts his wife most of the time but when he is in his more suspicious moods he gets very jealous. Although he trusts her in one sense he often wonders what she is doing during the day and makes frequent telephone calls to confirm she is still at home. Despite his suspicious nature once he makes friends they remain friends for life and he will do anything for them.

THE DEPENDENT TYPE

Miss Zeta is a fashion model. She wanted to be a ballet dancer when she was young but the strain of constant practice and physical exercise was too much for her and she drifted into modelling. She is glad she made the move and only regrets that her career cannot be a long one. At present she is attractive and gets a great deal of attention from male admirers. She has always liked being the centre of interest and her job satisfies these needs. She has always been good at acting and she is now so good at it that others wonder if she is acting all the time. If she is alone she gets bored easily and quickly looks for company again. She laughs and cries easily and is very sensitive to her surroundings. Although she has many boyfriends and would like to get married eventually, she finds it hard to choose between them. The young men that interest her most are usually unreliable but the dependable boyfriend she always turns to in times of difficulty bores her at other times. She relies on other people a great deal and the thought that worries her most is to be alone in the world.

THE FUSSY TYPE

Mr Eta is a senior official in a local government department. He prides himself on his conscientiousness and reliability. He has never been late for work in thirty years and people say they might as well set their watches by his arrival time as he is more punctual than any clock. He likes everything to run according to a set routine and his department runs like clockwork. He does not like change and if asked to take on an entirely new problem is put out at first because he has no rules to follow. He dresses soberly and conventionally and is formal in his social relationships. He likes to plan ahead as far as possible so that his future is predictable. In his spare time he collects stamps and coins, and these are beautifully ordered and presented. He cannot understand the haphazard ways in which young people run their lives and gets irritated with his teenage children for having no plans for the future and dressing in sloppy clothes. He is a great believer in authority and complains there is not enough of it in modern society. He lives in a neat house in a quiet suburb and has respectable neighbours who share his views. His garden is exceptionally well looked after although some feel he tries too hard to make his lawn look like a bowling green and his impeccable display of bedding plants – wallflowers in the spring, petunias and marigolds in the summer – might sometimes be changed for something new.

These personality pen-portraits are too short to get anything more than a glimpse of the types of people they

39

represent, and whole books could be written about each of them. Nevertheless I think you should have little difficulty in identifying people you know in one or more of the descriptions and may recognize yourself in the example of the personality type you obtained from the questionnaire. You may have some difficulty in accepting the picture of yourself painted by the example, but remember that each one is a stereotype. The people of this world cannot be put into seven groups only, but they share many characteristics. You should at least recognize some aspects of yourself in one of the types I have described. Once you have decided on your personality type, stick to it, even if the fit is far from perfect, because this will be needed in the exercise we are carrying out later.

How is stress related to these personality types? The most impressive differences are found between the driving successful (Mr Alpha) and placid easy-going personality (Mr Beta). Research in the United States over many years has shown that the Mr Alphas of this world are two to five times more likely than Mr Betas to get heart disease. If we accept that heart disease can be the result of prolonged harmful stress it is easy to see how the driving, aggressive, successful person is more likely to be stressed. He goes around looking for change which creates more demands on mind and body. He never relaxes and even when he has achieved one target in life he sets himself another, usually one that is even more demanding. What is unfortunate is that each success in life encourages him to strive still harder. One way in which our society creates unnecessary stress is by excessively praising success in every walk of life, and making out that if you are not a success you must automatically be a failure. Most advertising slogans shout at you to become successful – or perish in mediocrity. 'You too can be successful at work and with the opposite sex; you too can earn enough money to pay for all the goodies we want you to buy; you too can have a marvellous memory, be self-confident, look twenty years younger than you are, be the envy of your friends.' If you stop to think about these claims you will realize they cannot be true. If it was really so easy to achieve these aims then everyone would be successful, and if everyone is successful the word loses its meaning. In W. S. Gilbert's words: 'If everyone is somebody, then no one's anybody.' All success is bred on competition, and there can only be a few winners. Where our society has a lot to answer for is in its adulation of the winner. Once he has won he has to go on winning, and if he falters in the slightest he is abandoned as a failure. Our personalities are partly moulded by the environment in which we live, and although our driving successful Alphas may destroy themselves, they are encouraged to do so by society. They rise to the top of national and multinational organizations, make them more efficient so they make bigger profits. More money can be invested to make the organization bigger so it can employ more people and produce more. By producing and selling more everyone's standard of living is raised and the country becomes more prosperous.

So although you probably read the description of Mr Alpha with distaste and recognized none of your own characteristics in him, he is the most favoured personality type in our Western society. I am sure you have wished that you were more like him at some time in your life, particularly when you have come across a problem and not had the stamina or will to overcome it. Much of our lives is governed by Alpha principles laid down by society. The Peter principle, named after a Canadian who first described it, says that people at work are promoted till they reach the level of incompetence. To begin with they are in junior low-paid posts, but as they master these they are promoted to senior ones. As each new post is tackled and overcome new horizons beckon, until at last a post is attained which is just too much to cope with. This is the peak of occupational success and obviously varies from person to person. Unfortunately this post is often the most stressful of them all, because it makes demands on us that cannot be compensated for. We are playing the success–stress game without realizing it.

When we read about business executives with ulcers, heart disease, high blood pressure and other diseases of stress we naturally think that their jobs are the prime cause of their troubles. But this is far too simple. We select the driving, successful personalities for the important executive posts, because these personalities are the only ones that can cope with them. Of course, once they are in such posts, their personalities are allowed full scope of expression and stress is increased. Unfortunately too many jobs require the same qualities of energy, drive, competitiveness, intense self-discipline and desire to succeed. Although this demand seems to be creating more Alphas in our midst – evidence suggests there are more in America than in Great Britain – far too many of us are encouraged to believe we have these qualities when we lack them. If we take such jobs we are like square pegs in round holes, stress and conflict increases and we suffer unnecessarily. So do not give in too readily to demands that you should 'make a success of your life' and take on a life-style that is quite alien to you.

To keep harmful stress to a minimum your personality needs to be matched to your life-style. We just need to look at the way our different personality types cope with the same external situation to realize why stress affects each of us in a different way. Imagine asking each of our seven personalities to make a speech on a subject of his or her choice to a group of people. Mr Alpha would have no problem in public speaking and would produce an impressive, driving and polished speech, but it would have to be fitted in with many other demands on his time. Mr Beta would probably not prepare a speech at all and give a fireside chat. Miss Gamma would be thrown into a panic at the thought of public speaking and do her utmost to get out of the task, as would Mr Epsilon who would hate to talk to so many strangers. On the other hand, Miss Zeta and Mr Delta would positively enjoy the occasion as it would add sparkle and novelty to the day. Mr Eta would take the occasion seriously and prepare his speech with great care, possibly practising in front of a mirror beforehand to make sure he looks and sounds the part. While the exercise of standing up in public and talking in a way that makes reasonable sense is bound to have some stressful elements, the main difference between those who do not mind public speaking and those who are troubled by it is that the latter group are stressed for a long time before, and sometimes after, the speaking. If we are asked to recall the most nervous part of speaking in public most of us would pick on the time immediately before we start speaking. This is the time when our mouths feel dry, our voices croak, our legs feel like jelly and we wish we were a hundred miles away. The thought of feeling like this would make Miss Gamma refuse to agree to the talk, as she would worry for weeks in advance and probably be paralysed by fright when the time came for the speech. While Mr Beta might be mildly stressed for twenty minutes during his talk, Miss Gamma would be afflicted by major stress for many weeks.

Another reason for stress affecting each of us differently is that the change it produces varies from one to another. Swimming a hundred metres is no problem for an experienced swimmer, but for someone who is unfit and rarely swims it is an ordeal that leaves him exhausted for the rest of the day. The stress of more ordinary change also shows similar variation. If each of our personality types was required to move house there would be a range of stress extending from Mr Delta, who is so used to moving he can do it while half asleep, to Mr Epsilon and Mr Eta who tend to stay in the same place whenever they have the choice. Of course personality matches behaviour, as the types who hate change keep it to a minimum, but it means that those who dislike a particular stress have the least experience of dealing with it.

Although we have remarkable abilities to overcome problems and adapt to strange situations we must not assume that man is superman. We may like or dislike our basic personalities but we cannot ignore them. We also cannot change them to a significant degree, at least not after the age of twenty-five. Social and mental engineers sometimes have visions of a future when personality can be changed to order. Just imagine what a terrible world that would be. We might choose to be super-efficient successful people like Mr Alpha but with no one to control or supervise, a country of Prime Ministers with no people to govern. Or if the power to change personality fell into the hands of a dictator we could be programmed to be dull, obedient slaves with no independent thoughts or actions. No, the variation in personality is too precious to be thrown away. Coming to terms with ourselves and accepting our strengths and weaknesses honestly is a necessary prelude to living with stress. This is not an easy task. 'O would some power the giftie gie us, to see ourselves as others see us,' wrote Robert Burns. Most of us do not have that power, but at least we can listen to what others have to say. Once we have accepted our personalities, warts and all, we can plan our lives in a sensible way.

4

How to Recognize Harmful Stress

In the second part of this book I shall be describing different ways of treating harmful stress. Harmful stress, which includes distress and strain, has no advantages and should be kept to a minimum, if not eliminated altogether. Rather than describe each of the ways of treating stress in neat little chapters I want you to come with me on a voyage of discovery. It is like one of the mystery tours beloved by coach operators in which the passengers have no idea of their destination when they board the bus. But in this case I want each reader to be a driver. The route will be decided by your personalities. Each personality type will take a different route, but I would like to think you will end up in destinations which have one thing in common: they are free from harmful stress. The reason for choosing this approach, which means that from now onwards you could read the rest of the book in any order, is our old chestnut, the individuality of stress. It is impossible to say that any one way of coping with stress is better than any other because not only do the causes differ, but also the people who show the effects of stress.

If you have any of the symptoms we have discussed in earlier chapters the question you need to ask is simply, are your symptoms getting better or worse? If they are getting worse your stress is not doing you any good and may be doing you harm. Unfortunately no one can put a time scale on stress, but in general we are talking about unpleasant feelings that have lasted for weeks or months when we refer to harmful stress, and if they are getting worse but have only lasted a day or so you can assume for the time being that they are healthy.

When it comes to distinguishing between mental stress and the normal ups and downs of life we are on difficult territory. In the last resort each individual has to decide the dividing line for himself. Some people can be under stress even though everything in their lives is satisfactory, at least in a material way. They have jobs which are interesting and in which they can go at their own pace, they are happily married with delightful children and are physically fit. Not a cloud seems to be visible in their personal skies but yet they can have all the symptoms of stress. Why? The reason is that their lives have no meaning. Nothing they do seems to matter and so they are troubled. Even if there is no obvious explanation for your feelings of dissatisfaction they can still be due to stress.

Detecting silent harmful stress is not an exercise you can easily do alone. Although you should be able to appreciate the symptoms of stress, you put a mental block on your awareness and pretend nothing is wrong. True, others may be constantly telling you to calm down and take less responsibility or may be suffering as a result of your response to stress, but you ignore them. I pointed out earlier that only you can judge the intensity of your own feelings, but others are in a better position to judge how they affect those around you. You might not be aware of any feelings of stress and only show it by making a misery of other people's lives. So if people are yearning for a time in the past when you were a nicer person to live with, or work for, or if you find that your friends are melting away and no longer seeking your company, perhaps you should think whether it is you rather than they they that have changed. The suspicious Epsilons among you will find this admission very difficult. It is surprising how often people can look back at times in their lives when they behaved out of character and be amazed that they failed to recognize the problems that now are transparently clear. You can avoid this by listening with more attention to the comments of people that you respect and not just dismissing them as ignorant criticisms.

I have chosen to separate your personalities in the routes you take through this book, because each type has a different susceptibility to stress. The ambitious Alphas are particularly liable to get the physical diseases of stress, the peptic ulcer, the coronary heart disease, migraine and high blood pressure. This group is in control of its emotions and mental stress is much less common. Feelings of anger, irritability, nervousness and depression are sometimes noticed but are quickly suppressed. They get in the way of success and progress and can be forgotten. The stress therefore has its main impact on the body. Our worrying Gammas are much more likely to have mental stress. The reactions of the sympathetic nervous system that we all feel occasionally happen so frequently with them that they seem to dominate life. These people are much less likely to develop the physical diseases of stress although they do so more often than the placid Betas. It may be an over-simplification but it appears that if stress can be expressed outwardly in the form of mental disturbance it is less likely to turn inwards and affect the body.

Placid types show the least harmful stress. This is predictable, because they are seekers of stability, not of change, and happiest when few demands are made on them. They experience less stress in all its forms, both healthy and harmful, than the other types and so suffer much less from its ill-effects. The other personality types have less clear-cut relationships with stress but there still are differences between them. The conscientious Etas who like to have the whole of life organized in advance suffer stress if they are repeatedly asked to adjust to changes that are beyond their control. Although they can show both mental and bodily stress they tend towards the latter. Their high principles and strong sense of duty often lead to greater stress than in other types of personality, as they will tolerate the intolerable for much longer. The carefree Deltas are closest to the placid Betas and have a much lower predisposition to harmful stress. But their need for variety and excitement leads them into many potentially harmful situations that others would not contemplate. Our illustration of Mr Delta described a man who liked parachute jumping but this is only one example of sought after stress. Deltas are more likely to have accidents because they take risks in all areas of life. They drive fast and recklessly and often seek out danger. They lack foresight and do things which fulfil their need for excitement because of the risks involved. It is unfortunate that they can only reach the extreme levels of excitement they crave by taking risks and courting disaster. The high wire artiste who performs incredible feats of agility eighty feet above the ground creates much more excitement for himself and his audience if he does not use a safety net. The Delta types are unwilling to derive all their excitement in the passive way of the spectator at the circus, race track or boxing ring and prefer to be actively involved.

The dependent Zetas and suspicious Epsilons are more likely to have the mental consequences of harmful stress, but under quite different circumstances. Zetas do not like being alone and any prolonged isolation will be highly unpleasant for them. They express their feelings readily, almost too readily for some people who wonder if they are exaggerated at times, and are likely to respond

48

to the ups and downs of life with appropriate displays of emotion. The Epsilons, on the other hand, prefer being alone and are most distressed when they are forced to rub shoulders with many people, particularly when there is no opportunity to avoid them. This stress, which is actively desired by the Zetas, is harmful to the Epsilons because it reinforces their worries and suspicions, and shows in both the mental and physical spheres. Such people prefer a few people around them whom they can trust absolutely; the rest of humanity are potential enemies.

Although most of the ingredients of a problem likely to produce harmful stress are unique there is an important contribution from personality. I emphasize again that we cannot change personality, so simple solutions to stress are just not realistic. Making everybody adopt the lifestyle of the placid Betas in our midst on the grounds that it would reduce stress would be quite wrong. This lifestyle would be incompatible with all the other personality types and therefore produce a host of new stresses. We noted earlier that everyone has an optimum level of stress at which they are most happy, and there are great differences in these levels between our personality types. Harmful stress can result if the level of stimulation becomes too low as well as too high.

Our personality types vary in the risk of getting harmful stress and the way in which it is usually shown. These are summarized on page 46, so that you can see at a glance how your own personality type fares.

We can now start the mystery tour. The first stage is easy and most of us will continue on the same route. The only ones who are going to be diverted are the anxious worrying types of personality we came across in the last chapter. If you are one of the people like Miss Gamma who has always been highly anxious I would like you to move straight on to Chapter 6. I emphasize that here I am only referring to people who have tended to be nervous all their lives and can never remember being any different. Others may have a very good reason for feeling anxious but at some time in the past before they were put under stress, they were not nervous. Nobody is under constant stress from the moment they are born to the time they die and so if you cannot recollect being calm and relaxed at any time in your life you must have the Gamma-type personality. There is some evidence that this personality type runs in families, so if you feel you are in this category I would be surprised if a close relative did not feel similarly.

All other personality types should continue to Chapter 5, no matter what type of stress they have been under and how long it has lasted. You will be going on your separate ways in due course so do not be concerned.

TYPE OF PERSONALITY	RISK OF HARMFUL STRESS	TYPE OF HARMFUL STRESS
(a) ambitious	very high	physical
(b) placid	very low	physical
(c) worrying	very high	mental
(d) carefree	low	physical
(e) suspicious	moderate	mental and physical
(f) dependent	moderate	mental
(g) fussy	moderate	physical

5

Survival of the Fittest

You probably recognize this expression. It was first used to describe Charles Darwin's theory of evolution, a theory proposed over a century ago. Darwin suggested that all living things developed from a common ancestor by a gradual process taking millions of years. Chance variation from one generation to the next accounted for all the differences in the animal and plant kingdoms. Most of these variations were of no long-term value and so the species died out – the most famous examples are the dinosaurs – but some of the changes were very useful because they made the animal or plant better suited to its surroundings. So it thrived and multiplied at the expense of other species. Such a series of chance variations, according to the theory, led to the emergence of the most successful species of them all, man. Man is successful because of his highly superior intelligence which not only helps him to defeat competitors but gives him the power to change and control his living conditions in a way granted to no other species, so that he is even better suited to his surroundings. So the phrase 'survival of the fittest' is well suited to man. The weak go to the wall and the strong survive.

What has this got to do with stress? A great deal. We go through exactly the same process in our daily lives. When we come across a problem we have two choices: we can solve or overcome it or we can avoid it. Better still, we organize a niche for ourselves in life which is so well suited to us that we do not come across serious problems at all. Which choice we take depends a great deal on our personalities. The driving successful type, the Alphas we came across earlier, are always looking for new heights to scale, new problems to solve, and are more concerned about changing their surroundings than living in harmony with them. These are the people who are most prone to the diseases of stress because they deliberately put themselves under pressure and are only happy when they are in the thick of things. If you are this type of personality you are not going to change this pattern of living because it would be completely out of character. Your best policy is to concentrate on controlling the harmful effects of stress by one of the techniques described in the next chapter. You can move straight on to Chapter 6 now if you wish.

But of course this is not the best way of dealing with stress because you are only lessening the stress rather than removing it. There are many others who may on the surface be like the driving Alpha types but their basic personalities are quite different. They are forced by outside pressures to drive themselves harder than they would like; they are controlled by rather than controlling their lives. The trouble is that the more successful they are the more the pressures crowd in. Almost every day we can pick up a newspaper and read that some household name, a politician, pop star, sportsman or entertainer has succumbed to stress in one form or another. Yet another overdose has been taken, or the star's personal physician has advised complete rest because of 'severe strain', or the entertainer has broken down on stage. Once carried away by the system of success it is difficult to escape except through illness. Success so often means keeping up an image, which really means living a lie. The face the public sees is not your real face, it is a plastic face fashioned by the publicity men, all of whom grow fat on your success while it destroys you.

Perhaps the best people to cope with this type of stress are those who from birth onwards are in the public eye, such as members of the Royal Family. At least if you spend all your years in the glare of publicity you are more likely to adapt to the pressures that it brings. For others who have the misfortune to have fame thrust upon them the important thing is to keep your public and private faces as natural as possible. Even the best actor sometimes has an off day and the strain of a role that goes against your true self will eventually grind you down.

You may feel I am painting too gloomy a picture of success. My concern is with uncontrolled success in any part of life, be it at work, at leisure or in relationship with others. We all need an element of success in life to maintain our self-esteem, and, provided it is not exploited too much, this can bring rewards without harmful stress. We also need to be reminded that failure can also be very stressful. The failure of the jilted lover, the bankrupt tycoon and the unsuccessful examination candidate is so often stressful because pride is hurt. Sometimes the blow is too hard to bear and suicide is seen as the only way out of the conflict. The highest rate of suicide this century was not, as you might expect, during the horrifying stresses of war, but in peace-time, during the Great Depression (a very apt name) following the economic collapse in 1929. Those who were the most well off had more to lose and many committed suicide rather than face the indignity of abandoning their way of life. They all felt some personal responsibility for their financial ruin even when it was caused by factors beyond their control. When similar destruction to property and living standards was caused by the Blitz in the Second World War the people who suffered felt no personal responsibility for their plight. Suicide fell to the lowest level for many years but the stress still wreaked its damage and the number of peptic ulcers shot up alarmingly.

But in our present affluent society we seldom come across such severe stresses that are quite beyond our control. As we noted earlier, we have a choice of actions. Of course, the very fact of having a choice can produce its own share of stress, as often we cannot decide between conflicting interests. Many have commented on the eerie calm of the man sentenced to death in the minutes before his execution, but of course at this time there is no personal choice left, and stress is much less than earlier, when perhaps he entertained some hope of reprieve.

In making this choice it is helpful to bear in mind what we said earlier about the survival of the fittest. The best choice is one which leads to the best match of you and your surroundings. When Darwin first proposed his theory he used the phrase 'survival of the adapted' and only later was 'adapted' changed to 'fittest'. Adapted is a much better word because it includes all the ways in which you can cope with the problems of stress, while 'fittest' suggests that only drive and aggression will succeed. It is only when you have adapted that the changes at the heart of stress are overcome.

If you can successfully adapt you have by far the best 'cure' for your stress. Of course it is not a 'cure' in the real sense because you have removed the cause rather than treated the disease. Although on the surface this appears less glamorous than curing your stress with some special treatment it is much better because if it is done properly the stress will not come back. But like most things in life the best approach is the one which needs the most work. It is much easier to pretend that stress-related disease is not a personal but a medical problem, because this means you can absolve yourself from responsibility. If the treatment you receive fails in any way you can blame others instead of yourself, and if it succeeds, you have been told what to do rather than working out the solution for yourself. There are no easy answers to the problems caused by stress, each personal stress has unique qualities and the ideal treatment is also unique, carefully fashioned for that problem alone.

It is still possible to give guidance on the ways to go about adapting to harmful stress. We have to remember that to adjust successfully we must bear our basic personalities in mind, because we can make what appears to be a marvellous adjustment at first but if it conflicts with our basic personalities it will soon rebound on us. The driving ambitious type who decides to opt out of his job as head of an international combine and go back to nature in the back of beyond may at first be relieved. But before long his competitive urges will be rekindled and he will only be happy if he can organize the rural community in the same way as he did his former company. There are suggestions that some of those who left highly paid jobs in London and other major cities and joined crofting communities in the north of Scotland are having just this problem. The simple local crafts bring in a little money which is enough to live on, but our ambitious type is not satisfied by this. He sees the opportunities for mass production and improved sales by advertising, and before long the crofting community is another big business. (This is the second opportunity for any driving ambitious personalities who are still with us to move on to Chapter 6.)

We so often let harmful stress get out of control because of blind spots in our make-up which stop us from seeing the obvious solution. Let us look at some typical examples of this among the personality types we came across earlier.

Mr Beta, we will recall, is placid, good-natured and

perhaps a little lazy. In general he is protected from stress but like many placid people he enjoys food. Unfortunately people who enjoy food and do not take a great deal of exercise are liable to eat more than their bodies need. So Mr Beta gets fat. He does not admit to himself that he eats too much or is fat, but he agrees with his close friends that he has 'a weight problem' (this is so much nicer than saying you are too fat). He wonders whether this may be something to do with his glands and visits the doctor, who examines him and tells him bluntly he is overweight and so must be eating too much. Mr Beta cannot believe this. He never eats between meals and although he enjoys his food he has never been greedy. When it is pointed out that his meals are three times bigger than those of other members of his family and his penchant for cakes and buns makes it more likely for him to put on weight he protests how little food they contain because they are light and full of air. If he takes no notice and stays too fat, he will get tired easily, feel depressed because he is not able to do so much, and have many arthritic aches and pains. These symptoms are all due to him carrying round a body that is 50 per cent heavier than his frame is built for. It may take him many months to accept the simple fact that he is eating too much, and that fat cannot come out of thin air. One reason he finds it so difficult is that eating plays so important a part in his life. He is hospitable, sociable and generous and food is involved in many of his activities. Once food is established as one of the good things of life it is very difficult to accept it can do harm. But if he can come to terms with his problem and realize it can be overcome by proper dieting, either through his own efforts or through the assistance of an organization such as Weight-watchers, and if the dieting can be achieved without the addition of pills or other medical forms of treatment, it is much more likely to be successful in the long run.

Mr Epsilon and other suspicious personality types usually produce different stress problems. In fact they are frequently thin and underweight. In days of old they might have employed food tasters to test each meal and make sure that it was not poisoned! The niche which suits Mr Epsilon is a small one and he quickly gets under stress if moved out of it. For instance, the headmaster of his school may feel that Mr Epsilon's many years of devoted service to teaching should be rewarded by making him deputy headmaster. This is accepted gratefully by Mr Epsilon who is glad that his true worth has been recognized. His duties involve much less teaching children and more with organizing the school curriculum. When taken away from the children with whom he feels secure Mr Epsilon gets more suspicious. He spends most of his time with other teachers, discussing and co-ordinating their work. Occasionally, and inevitably with this type of work, there are minor disagreements. Mr Epsilon inflates these to major crises in his own mind and every criticism is seen as a personal attack. He feels the other staff are all against him and are plotting his downfall. He cannot concentrate on his work and it naturally suffers. I need not go any further as you can predict the consequences unless the stress is removed. Mr Epsilon should never have accepted or have been offered the deputy headmaster post. He should be rapidly restored to his old position, or moved to a similar one in another school if the damage to his relationships has gone too far.

Those of us who need people to the extent of depending on them like Miss Zeta are more likely to come across harmful stress in close relationships. Such people need attention and variety in life but are often troubled by insecurity. So Miss Zeta might be very tempted to marry her dependable boyfriend, one of the few signs of constancy in her life. This may be right for her but it is equally likely to be wrong. If he is interested in settling down and leading a more predictable life, conflict lies ahead. Miss Zeta needs the attention of her many admirers and the excitement of her job, which takes her to many different countries. The change to a quieter life, particularly if she gives up her job and has children, will be too great for her to bear, and as it conflicts with her personality, she may never adapt to it. So the cycle of marital stress will begin. The temptation to start extramarital affairs with her old flames will be strong and the boredom of a life-style which is wholly alien to the novelty she is used to will be too much to bear. She introduces novelty by neglecting her wifely duties, gadding about the country seeking new adventures, and comes into increasing conflict with her husband. Even if he is quiet, tolerant and good-natured, she may create arguments just to satisfy her need for variety, as fighting with him will be more interesting than the serenity of domestic bliss. If he is not jealous she will make sure she makes him so, and soon the marriage will be on the road to destruction.

Of course there are many reasons for marriages going wrong and it would be wrong to blame them all on personality clashes. In Miss Zeta's case the solution is likely to involve a major change in her role in the marriage. She is not a home-loving domesticated dutiful wife, who is happy to stay on her own all day and spend quiet evenings with her husband. Her personality demands variety and people around her. She needs to come to some arrangement with her husband so that her independence can be maintained. Perhaps she could return to work or arrange other activities that can satisfy the needs of her personality and allow her to appreciate the value of her husband without feeling tied down. Although marital stress can have dozens of causes there are really only two solutions: the marriage breaks up, or the parties adjust their attitudes so that they live together in harmony again. The worst way of coping is to accept it as a fact of life and do nothing about it. This is often justified 'for the sake of the children' and other equally noble motives but it should not be accepted as the only solution.

By now you will be getting into the swing of things and could probably predict the changes that would lead to harmful stress in the carefree Mr Delta. This personality type likes variety, is impulsive, sometimes a little childish, and rather vain. Because Mr Delta has little foresight and is prone to flattery it is easy to see how success could turn sour on him. Suppose a national broadcasting company was to discover hidden talents in him and make him a disc jockey with his own show, or set him up as a front man with a chat programme. He would receive instant popularity (in this day and age this is absolutely predictable) but instead of putting this in perspective, he would be convinced that he was really a great guy. His life would lose all semblance of control. He would get involved in complicated personal relationships with his female fans, his working and leisure time would be a whirl of continual change with no time for reflection, and he would overreach himself as vanity gradually replaced common sense. The cycle of success gets out of hand and the stress will finally surface as drug abuse or overdosage, alcoholism, or the ultimate humiliation, a breakdown while 'on the air'. Dealing with this type of stress in Mr Delta is a difficult problem. He and success do not mix and if he is unfortunate enough to become a star his best hope is to have a good agent who will protect him from the publicity that would otherwise destroy him.

The anxious worrying types will not be reading this

chapter so we can exclude an example of Miss Gamma under stress. Unfortunately virtually every change that is any way out of the ordinary is going to have its damaging effects on her. So we move on to our final type, fussy Mr Eta. As we noted earlier, this type is highly organized and tries to keep change to a minimum by adjusting to it in advance. But many changes are beyond his control. He likes his peace and quiet and although he can tolerate a fair amount of bustle and activity it becomes disturbing if it interferes with his routines. If his quiet house and garden was to change from being a desirable residential area because it was in the flight path of an airport he would begin to have problems. The continual roar of air-craft overhead and the increased bustle of activity round his home would be disturbing, although he would be less inclined to move house than other personality types be-cause of his dislike of change. But if the excessive noise and activity increases he will lose control. We need to remind ourselves that excessive noise and overcrowding are not natural to us, and although we may often choose to live in a city because it is close to our work and has a better range of shopping, entertainment and other facili-ties than the country, it is far from being the ideal sur-roundings.

Man is a social being and lives best in groups, but not when they are very large. Too many people packed into too small a space becomes stressful for everybody. When other animals get overcrowded in this way they get short of food and large numbers leave the group, even when the alternatives are far from attractive. You have prob-ably heard of the lemming, a small animal rather like a vole, which responds to overcrowding by mass emigra-tion. Thousands of lemmings will file into the sea from an overcrowded island and only a handful survive to reach new land. We do not have the same sensitivity to overcrowding and unfortunately the drift to the cities is continuing in almost all countries of the world. Because stress follows change and because the amount and speed of change is so much greater in cities than the country-side, all problems of stress are greater. Those who live in small towns or rural surroundings will live on the aver-age nearly five years longer than those in cities, where there are also more diseases of harmful stress. Although Mr Eta would be disinclined to make a move because of his unwillingness to make big changes in his life, he will suffer if he decides to stay, unless he can band together with like-minded residents in his suburb and persuade the authorities that the proposed changes are detrimental to their quality of life, and should be aban-doned or channelled elsewhere.

Obviously we could go on indefinitely conjuring up scenes from the lives of these personalities that would be unpleasantly stressful for some and have no effect on others, but I hope the general message is clear. The ideal way of dealing with harmful stress is to neutralize it in exactly the same way in which healthy stress is overcome. The resources needed to cancel out stress are often con-siderable, and it may be a long haul. But we often fail to overcome stress properly because we adopt old ways of dealing with it. Most of the time our minds run along well ordered grooves like the wheels of a tram and this protects us from a lot of unnecessary stress. But harmful stress only develops when these grooves are no longer right for us and we have to make new ones. This means thinking, and thinking means hard work. But until we recognize the problem we will never find the solution. When we recognize the symptoms of stress it is much easier to rush off and try one of the treatments for stress described in later chapters than it is to ponder a little and work out why we feel as we do. It is also much more difficult to remove the problem than to treat the symptoms directly. All the pressures are on us to take the easy way out and try the latest treatment for stress. We shall find they are not as impressive as they appear to be and can never cure stress. This needs repeating, particularly as we are constantly being assailed by the latest and best of anti-stress treatments, which so often claim to cure but never can.

In removing harmful stress we come back time and time again to the paramount importance of balancing our internal needs with the pressures from outside. So many of our lives today are highly specialized because society demands experts in everything. But a balanced society in which every member has a specialized role produces a lot of highly unbalanced individuals. The professor who is trained to teach, write and develop new knowledge is not encouraged to treat his illnesses, mend his plumbing when it springs a leak, or service his own car. All these jobs are done by other experts who require special training, so that life becomes chopped up by hundreds of demarcation lines, each special task needing a solution from someone other than ourselves. But the professor is not just a walking brain, much as society may like him to be, and his body and mind require the same balance of activities as the rest of humanity. In talking about the survival of the adapted in our present age we should not just take the artificial goals set by society as the ones we should be aiming for, but include the whole of our lives. Although, as we have seen, people have different goals and require different levels of stress to keep in balance, they all have certain basic needs. 'Do you feel fit?' is perhaps the simplest way of deciding whether you are under harmful stress or have any form of illness. Fitness includes both physical and mental well-being and can only be attained by proper use of our bodies and minds. If you never take any exercise apart from walking to the station or pushing the vacuum cleaner over the floor you cannot be physically fit. You will feel so much better if you take more exercise. Of course if you have spent many years being underactive and overweight some damage may already have been done and you would be advised not to take activity too strenuously. Every winter there are a disquieting number of deaths following heavy snowfalls when people have to dig the snow away from around their cars. For those unfamiliar with exercise the result is often a heart attack with fatal consequences. Just in the same way that a mind which is never asked to think will produce tension and anxiety when forced to work out a problem, a body that is allowed to grow flabby with disease will fail when asked to take on a physical task. This is not to say we should all be Tarzans and Janes swinging through the trees in a self-indulgent display of muscular prowess but Western society in general is physically unfit and needs to be reminded of it. Our Victorian forefathers recognized the value of keeping a balance between work, rest and play and although at times they were a little rigid in the application of their philosophy we could do with a dose of it nowadays.

If you think that you are suffering from harmful stress I would like to think that after finishing this chapter you will know what is causing it and already have some idea how you are going to rid yourself of it. The most successful among you will not need any of the special aids described later, because you will be able to put yourselves back into balance through your own efforts. This does not mean that success will come immediately. Often you may be inhibited from taking the right corrective action because in the short-term it appears to be wrong. Nobody likes to stop eating when they feel hungry, or ask for demotion because it means a big drop in income, but if you never take the first step you will be stuck indefinitely. You will also have realized from this chapter that how others have coped with their stresses may be quite irrelevant to your problem, and any advice you take should be from people whom you know well and whose judgement you respect. In any case you are going to have to make the final decision in the end no matter how many people advise you on the way.

If you think you have learnt nothing from this chapter and cannot wait to read on to some straight talk about treating stress directly, then by all means move on. But this attitude implies that you already know why you are suffering from stress but have done nothing to remove it. This may be true, but we tend to assume it is true when change is possible. As we live in a world of change there is no reason why you should be exempt. So why wait for a crisis to show the way of overcoming your stress? If you are right in fully appreciating why you are suffering, it is ridiculous to accept a second-best treatment if you have any possibility of removing or lessening the cause. I am confident that all the placid Betas among you will be able to do this successfully, but first of all they should read Chapter 10. Some others will also be able to conquer their stress without any special help, but all the rest should come with me to Chapter 6.

6

Self-Control

Before we go into the details of controlling harmful stress through our own efforts we should recap on progress so far. We are assuming that you cannot banish stress from your lives either because you are such a worrying type that everything is stressful, or because you cannot find the cause of your stress, or that you know the cause only too clearly but can do nothing about removing it. Whatever the reason, the stress is harmful because it is with you continuously. The first part of treatment is to break into this cycle where the sympathetic nervous system and other hormones of stress have a completely free hand, and replace it with relaxation, so that you no longer feel anxious and worried, your muscles are no longer tense, and your heart and breathing rate slow to a regular resting level. When you are well you have no problem in relaxing but when under continual stress it needs a lot of work to earn a few moments of calm.

But there are techniques of relaxation that will help to make these moments longer. Read and follow the instructions below and you will understand the principles behind these techniques. It needs practice before you can relax fully at will and it is a good idea to start when you are already fairly relaxed. So for maximum effect follow the instructions after you have had a hot bath or feel tired after a hard day of physical work.

Tense the muscles of your right hand by making a fist. Hold this tension for half a minute. If you feel your grip relaxing tighten the fist still further. Slowly let the muscles relax and open out the hand and fingers. If your hand still feels tense make a fist again. Slacken the fist gradually till the hand is quite floppy and relaxed. Tense the arm and shoulder by bending the elbow and bringing your hand up against your shoulder. Hold this position for at least a minute. Each muscle in your arm will feel tight and stiff but when you let them relax they feel heavier and more comfortable.

Tense and relax the muscles of your left hand and arm in the same way. It should take less time to relax than the right arm but continue until both arms are quite loose. Move on to the muscles of your neck and face. Exercise these muscles by raising and lowering your eyebrows, putting your head right back and then bringing it down until your chin rests against your chest. Frown and relax your forehead alternately. Open and close your mouth and clench your teeth tightly together. Relax your jaw gradually and feel the tension go. Relax your neck and face so that all the muscles feel soft and smooth. Expand your chest by taking a deep breath and holding it for a few seconds. Slowly breathe out and feel the chest muscles relax. Take another deep breath and continue breathing slowly and deeply, slowly and deeply.

As you continue breathing deeply you will find it easier to relax all the muscles in your arms, chest, neck and face. Now lift your right leg off the ground with the knee held straight, hold it up for a few seconds and then slowly lower it to the ground. Do the same with the left leg. Continue doing this until your legs feel so tired and heavy that they seem to sink into the ground when they are relaxed. As your legs get more relaxed it becomes difficult to lift them up. Let them rest and feel the tension flowing away. Make sure that your feet, ankles and knees are completely relaxed as well before you let your legs rest completely.

Remember to continue your deep breathing while you

relax further. Each time you breathe out your muscles will relax a little more. Feel your body sinking down and getting heavier as you continue breathing more deeply. Let your back and stomach muscles relax as you breathe and feel a warm glow of relaxation pass over your whole body. Every muscle should now feel relaxed and your mind completely calm. Close your eyes and let the feeling of relaxation take over. Try and open your eyes again. It is not worth the effort; your lids are too heavy and you do not want to disturb your relaxation. Outside pressures no longer trouble you and you feel cut off from the world. Nothing troubles you now you are completely calm, completely calm and relaxed.

You are bound to feel more relaxed now if you have followed these instructions to the letter, but you will have to practise repeatedly before you get the full benefit. Once you have mastered the technique when you are already quite relaxed it is time to move on and learn to relax when you are feeling tense and strung up. Do not give up at this stage if at first the technique does not seem to be working. It takes time and application and often progress is made in fits and starts. Just when you feel that nothing has been achieved the principles of the technique will suddenly click and you are on your way.

Because the art of relaxation is so sought after in our modern world people have searched for bigger and better ways of achieving it. This is why there has been so much interest in yoga, transcendental meditation and other Eastern philosophies. These are really concerned with a way of life and it is difficult to transpose them to our Western society without losing a great deal. Nevertheless, the relaxation techniques of these philosophies have been modified so that they can be practised on their own without the subject necessarily taking on their religious beliefs and life-styles. They are probably not so effective when used in isolation in this way but they have become increasingly popular over the last few years. I am not an expert on yoga and transcendental meditation and there are very few Western doctors who can claim to be. So I am not able to pronounce on the best form of these treatments for stress. But as far as producing relaxation is concerned they are just more complicated forms of relaxation training.

For example, in transcendental meditation, which was founded by Maharishi Mahesh Yogi as a form of yoga, the aim is to concentrate on a thought in such a way that the thought itself disappears and the 'source of the thought' is reached. This difficult task can only be achieved by repeating a personal mantra, a ritual word which helps to drive other thoughts out of the mind, during meditation. The meditator's concentration is directed entirely to this mental search but as it involves cutting out all other stimulation it automatically leads to muscular relaxation, a slower heart beat and more regular breathing. Other techniques involve more complicated rituals but all achieve the same end if successful.

Special types of breathing are used in other forms of yoga so that air fills the bottom of the lungs first, and the proportion of time spent breathing in and out is also carefully regulated. Although it is possible to learn these techniques from books most people find it more helpful to be taught by those with special knowledge. There is likely to be an evening or day-time class teaching yoga and relaxation near where you live and it does no harm to enquire and enrol. If you cannot make much headway with relaxation training alone you could find yoga quite a different proposition, so do not be disheartened. There are lots of variations between the techniques and although there is little to choose between them it is best to stick to the same one rather than chopping and changing.

Once you become an expert you can reach a degree of mind control that you never even suspected. This will help you to 'blank your mind' when the pressures of stress become too much. Just think of the advantages of having this ability. Instead of bringing all the troubles of the day home in the evening so that they prevent your attempts to relax, you turn the 'job switch' off and forget them till the next morning. A very few people can even learn the trick of switching off whenever they feel themselves getting over-stressed, so the man who feels nervous about giving a speech to a large audience goes to sleep for five minutes beforehand, or someone like Miss Gamma who cannot get off to sleep at night carries out her relaxation exercises until she naturally drops off. But this ideal degree of control is rare. It takes time to develop full relaxation and many can only do it if they are in the right mood. It is most useful in putting a stop to stressful reactions that otherwise would reinforce themselves.

Hypnosis can also be used to aid relaxation, but is sometimes made out to be a more powerful treatment than it really is. Under hypnosis you are more suggestible and better able to respond to instructions telling you to relax. This of course requires a hypnotist, who issues the instructions whilst you are in the suggestible frame of mind. In deep hypnosis you can be so relaxed that you appear to be in a coma, but in fact you are still awake. Unfortunately only a small number of people make excellent hypnotic subjects and most of us cannot reach this state. But very few are completely unresponsive to hypnotic suggestion and it certainly helps us to relax further. Although at first a hypnotist may be needed to introduce us to the subject and illustrate the power of suggestion, later we can use the technique on ourselves through auto-hypnosis. If we feel relaxed when someone else is telling us to relax in a special way there is no reason why we ourselves should not do the telling. Some of my readers, particularly the Miss Zetas who depend on people, may find this hard to believe, but there is nothing especially potent in the person of the hypnotist; his power lies in your belief in him and to a lesser extent in what he says. So before long you can get the same beneficial effects by repeating instructions to yourself or by listening to an audiotape.

There are many ways of bringing the pleasures of relaxation home to you and I trust one of the ones I have described will be successful. I suggest the basic relaxation training first of all, yoga or transcendental meditation second, and only move on to hypnosis if these fail. The main reason for suggesting this order is financial. Relaxation training and yoga are cheap to learn or cost nothing at all, but hypnotists are expensive by comparison. Some have special skills at teaching relaxation and it is always better to choose one through the recommendation of a friend rather than picking one at random.

If you are successful in controlling harmful stress by relaxation you need go no further, although it may still be worth your while thinking about its cause. If the cause is still nagging away you will continue to be troubled even though you have an effective weapon to combat it at your disposal. There are other possible consequences. You may feel completely relaxed after trying the techniques but the pain or ache you thought was due to stress is still there. If this happens with any symptom, whether it is physical or mental, it is reasonable to assume that it is not due to stress or, if it is, that it has gone beyond the realm of psychological control and is now part of an illness. Relaxation is often a good diagnostic test. If you have severe pain in your back and find it remains exactly the same even when you have systematically relaxed every muscle group in your body, then your pain is unlikely to be due to the tension of stress. Your muscles may be in spasm for many other reasons or the pain may really be an internal one that feels as though it is on the surface even though it comes from inside the body. If you still suspect that your symptoms have a physical basis after you have got to this stage then it is wise to see your doctor about it. Seeing your doctor may be the next stage for others in our mystery tour. This will particularly apply to those who make absolutely no progress with relaxation training or other techniques and angrily discard them as a waste of time. Our driving ambitious and anxious worrying personalities are most likely to be in this position and, if so, should move on to the next chapter. If they make a little progress with relaxation but find that they cannot develop it further, then they can move ahead to Chapter 8. The other personalities should proceed as follows. The suspicious Epsilons and fussy Etas should also go to Chapter 8, but the dependent Zetas and carefree Deltas should go to Chapter 9, although the Zetas would be well advised to remind themselves of the message in Chapter 4 again first. Placid types who still feel under stress should go to Chapter 10, but I think they will be few. If you move on to any of the next four chapters you are admitting to yourself that you cannot solve your harmful stress on your own or by using advice from friends and relatives. You are moving on to the unknown world in which experts, some real and some self-appointed, suggest treatment of some kind. Although it is a strange land it is useful to know something of the terrain in advance so that misunderstanding can be kept to a minimum.

7

Doctor, I Can't Go on Like This

The family doctor is the expert who is most frequently approached by people suffering from harmful stress. Many years ago he and the parish vicar or priest were the only ones who were available. Now there are alternatives but a good doctor is often in the best position to advise you which is the most appropriate. Before going to see your doctor it is useful to have some idea about his likely knowledge of stress and disease. The general practitioner is, as the name implies, trained in general aspects of medicine rather than concentrating on one speciality. This does not mean he is not a specialist, for many illnesses such as the diseases of childhood, throat and chest infections, back pain, arthritis and migraine are treated much more often by the general practitioner than by the specialist, although once these conditions become serious hospital referral is necessary. So as stress is a common cause of disease your doctor is likely to have seen many people with problems similar to yours. But the average practitioner in the United Kingdom has about two and a half thousand people on his list and even if he had the ability to deal with all the problems caused by stress it would be quite impracticable for him to spend the necessary time as well as coping with all the other demands made on him. The average consultation with a general practitioner takes six minutes and so no time should be wasted in getting your problem over. The other point worth emphasizing is that the general practitioner is trained to identify physical disease more than mental illness. This is not because mental illness is uncommon in general practice, indeed it makes up more than a tenth of all consultations, but at least until recently, treatment was much more effective for physical disease and it is important not to miss diagnosing treatable disease. Harmful stress can be present in many forms and so it is no good saying to the doctor when he asks what is the matter that you are suffering from stress. That is about as informative as saying that you feel ill. Present your symptoms first and add any suggestions about their cause afterwards. Symptoms are changes in your bodily or mental function that you find unpleasant and different from your normal feelings. Try and describe them as accurately as possible and avoid jumping to the conclusion that they are due to stress. The first role of the doctor is to make a diagnosis, and this can only be done properly if he has all the relevant information in front of him. If your symptoms are physical ones he is likely to examine you to make sure that there are no abnormalities that could explain your symptoms in terms of known disease. If he is in any doubt about this he may arrange blood tests or other investigations and possibly refer you to a hospital.

If your symptoms are all in the mental sphere his options are more limited and may seem unsatisfactory to you. But put yourself in his place. You may be at the end of your tether because your marriage is breaking down, or you have just lost your job, or one of your children is seriously ill, or you have a court case pending. The list is endless, but all of these are problems that have no instant solution, otherwise you would not be sitting in his surgery. The doctor cannot solve the problem or take it away; all he can do is help you to live with it a little more comfortably. He may also be able to give you some sensible words of advice, particularly if he has known you and your family for a long time, but if he does say something which throws new light on the problem it is best to regard this as a bonus of his consultation rather than a right. He can also sympathize and reassure you and although both you and he realize that this is no solution it is comforting to know that someone can understand the difficulties you are going through at a deeper level than just recognizing that you have problems. But you cannot expect him to devote much time to this unless you are very lucky, so do not feel rejected or hard done by if your interview is ended more quickly than you would like.

The cry, 'I can't go on like this', is also a plea for more than sympathy. Prolonged and severe mental stress becomes mental agony and cannot be tolerated. The doctor has a way of reducing this degree of stress and making it more bearable. He can prescribe a tranquillizer. Tranquillizers are prescribed more often than any other class of drug in medicine and it helps to know something about them. First of all, do they work? Are they successful in reducing the effects of stress?

The answer is yes for most of the tranquillizers of today, but often no for the remedies of the past. The complicating factor is the 'placebo effect'. When a tablet or medicine is taken for any reason there is often an immediate feeling of relief long before the medicine has had any opportunity to be absorbed into the body. This is because we believe that we have taken something to help us and the very act of believing makes us feel better immediately. This effect is much greater if we have confidence in the person who has prescribed the medicine. Many years ago doctors had very little in the way of effective treatments. About the only common feature of medicines was that they tasted nasty, and it followed from Victorian logic that if something tasted unpleasant it must be doing good. But most of these medicines were placebos, and the doctors who prescribed them often realized it. They also realized that if they appeared to be highly knowledgeable men who seldom made mistakes and had a cure for every ill, they did far more good than if they appeared weak and ineffective. So they developed their omnipotent airs and were always careful to keep a certain distance from their patients so the element of mystery was maintained. Looking back on this you may feel it was deceitful and unfair to act in this way, but if you talk to elderly people about their attitude to doctors you will find that they often yearn for the old days when doctors were revered and could do no wrong.

Many of the old tranquillizers were placebos and whether or not they helped people depended on the doctor's charm and personality. Of course, if placebos cured people or permanently helped their symptoms doctors would be happy to prescribe them all the time. But unfortunately their effects seldom last longer than a few weeks. This may be quite satisfactory for some illnesses which are going to get better anyway, but those of you who think you have harmful stress are likely to have had symptoms for much longer.

One of the old tranquillizers that was far from being a placebo was alcohol in all its forms. Alcohol is a powerful tranquillizer, although those who have never drunk to excess might find this hard to believe. A small amount of alcohol may feel like a stimulant but this is an illusion, as it is really acting as a mild tranquillizer by first removing your inhibitions. In larger amounts it calms you down and if too much is drunk you will become unconscious. If you take alcohol for stress it seems to work, at least at first. You stop worrying about whatever it was that made you worry, you feel calm and relaxed, and you help yourself to another drink. The cycle has started, for one drink leads to another. When the effects of the alcohol wear off you are presented with the same problems that were there before you started drinking. So it is only natural to drink again to return to that happy land of make-believe where stress is a five-letter word with no meaning. Unfortunately alcohol is not just an escape from the problems of stress; it creates new ones and exacerbates those already present. The husband who does not get on with his wife and drowns his sorrows in the pub, the inefficient executive who removes his business worries at the bar of his club, the sportsman who fails to maintain his fitness yet boasts of his prowess in an alcoholic twilight world; they are all stereotypes from low budget movies, yet they all exist. The downward path started by alcohol abuse is painfully obvious to everyone else but the victim, who will blame all except drink for his plight. People under stress who are already moderate drinkers are the most likely to find themselves on the slope down to alcohol abuse. The temptation to take just that little bit more alcohol is very strong and the increased drinking pattern is established.

So alcohol is definitely out as a tranquillizer for combating stress? What of the others? Barbiturates used to be popular tranquillizers but they have exactly the same snags as alcohol. They tend to over-sedate, they impair judgement and they are addictive in regular dosage. Some people can get away with taking them regularly at night for insomnia without becoming hooked but those who take them during the day as well are almost bound to become addicted if they persist. As far as the brain is concerned, a barbiturate pill is the same as a large alcohol lozenge and the only reason there are many more alcohol addicts than barbiturate ones is that it is socially acceptable to drink alcohol, whereas barbiturates are only obtainable on prescription from doctors. In fact, doctors have become so concerned about barbiturate prescription because of their poor safety record and danger of addiction that they have tried to cut out their prescription altogether for the treatment of problems associated with stress.

The group of tranquillizers your doctor may consider prescribing is one which includes Librium, Valium and Mogadon, the trade names of drugs that are so commonly prescribed that almost everyone has heard of them. The reason your doctor will prefer these to the others is that they are much better at reducing anxiety and stress without seriously affecting other parts of the brain. So they can reduce the impact of stress without greatly impairing judgement and co-ordination. They are definitely not placebos. If you take a tablet it takes about an hour to get absorbed into the bloodstream and then it begins to act. You feel calmer and more confident, but if you have taken too large a dose you will feel sleepy. Of course if you are very nervous and only take a small dose you may notice nothing at all. The effects of one tablet last for about four hours, but if you take them regularly they can go on affecting you for over twenty-four hours. If you take one of these tablets regularly at night it is bound to affect you the next day as there is no such thing as the perfect sleeping tablet which just lasts for the night and is completely out of your system by morning.

What will a prescription for one of these drugs do for stress? Let us be clear first of all what it will not do. It will not remove the stress or alter it in any constructive way. It is in no way a substitute for the personal decisions to combat stress that we described earlier and will come to again later in this book. It will not give you sudden insight or understanding of the stress. People are getting to know more about the drugs they take and some of these statements may be obvious, but they are worth repeating. All a tranquillizer can do is to take the edge off your reaction to the stress and relieve your suffering. In case the word 'suffering' sounds a little strong, let me emphasize that it can be a great deal worse. Torture is often a more apt description for the mental reaction to a stress that just grinds on interminably like a dentist's drill into the brain. If stress is producing this kind of reaction it is ridiculous to deprive yourself of a tranquillizer because of strong principles that it is somehow wrong or a sign of weakness to take pills. By taking a pill when in this state you can at least lessen the stress on your mind and body and at best you allow yourself a breathing space which helps you to decide on the best way to remove the stress.

There are others who use tranquillizers in quite another way. They resort to taking them when they are not under severe stress at all. Quite often they are taken as an exercise in manipulation. The wife who is not getting on with her husband may make a visit to the doctor with the sole intention of getting a prescription for tranquillizers. She can then brandish her little bottle of pills in front of her husband and claim that he has 'driven' her to taking pills. This has less impact now than it used to, as so many people carry tranquillizers around with them, but if the ploy works the husband is shocked into examining his attitudes and behaviour. But the taking of pills is no indication of the amount of stress. Some will take them at the slightest whim, others will never do so.

It will be clear by now that if tranquillizers are being taken for stress they should only be taken occasionally, at times when the stress becomes unbearable. If you take them regularly there is a danger that you will take no further action to resolve the stress. You accept your lot as not a happy one, but the taking of tranquillizers makes it tolerable. But if you did not have them available the unpleasantness of the stress might drive you to do something about it, something constructive which might eventually remove the stress altogether. But there is another reason for not taking tranquillizers regularly. They can produce dependence and, rarely, addiction. This is not the same as addiction to alcohol or hard drugs but you can still get hooked. The first prescription is given for one or two weeks to tide over a crisis, but all too often it is repeated, not just once but dozens of times. The tranquillizer originally was like a crutch, to help you keep going while your emotions were repaired, but now you cannot live without them. When the tablets are stopped for any reason you feel nervous and tense again, and back you go for another prescription. But if you continue taking the tablets in the same dose for months or years your body gets used to them. A dose which used to knock you out when you first started the tablets now has virtually no effect and you have to increase the amount to keep you feeling calm. Some of our personality types are more likely to go this way than others. The Gamma types have felt nervous all their lives and it is not surprising that they turn to tranquillizers as a duck takes to water. They go on taking the pills because all life is stressful for their constitutions and anything which reduces their nervousness is going to be in demand. But it is much better to choose one of the techniques in the last chapter to reduce anxiety because there are fewer problems with repeated yoga and relaxation training than with repeated swallowing of tranquillizers. The dependent Zetas have been guided to this chapter last because they too are more likely to get hooked. Not only do they tend to rely on other people but also on medicines. Even if there is no need to go on taking them after the first prescription they feel lost without them and demand more. It is even possible for them to become dependent on dummy pills in exactly the same way, so the problem is in the mind rather than in the pills. So if you come into either of these types be very careful about taking tranquillizers and certainly try and avoid taking them regularly.

There are many other tablets used to treat problems caused by mental stress and it is wrong to assume they are all tranquillizers. There are stimulants and anti-depressants which act in quite a different way. Some are habit forming and some are not, some work immediately, others have a delayed effect, some are dangerous when taken with other drugs and certain foods, others are quite safe. Just as doctors can give different tablets for diseases of different parts of the body, they can give different medicines for the many mental reactions to stress, so do not assume that all tranquillizers are the same. Sometimes people get upset when they are given a tablet for nerves as they are convinced their bodies alone are reacting abnormally. If you have ever been in this position you will know the feeling; you feel slighted because your evidence has apparently been considered unreliable and your judgement wrong. But although such feelings are understandable they are unnecessary. We need reminding that the mind and body are not as separate countries linked only by radio and telephone communication, but are more like close relatives living and working together; almost everything that influences the mind will also influence the body, and vice versa. So a tranquillizer will not only reduce anxiety but also lower the blood pressure a little, lessen sweating and take away pains in the stomach by relaxing the muscles in the gut. It tells the sympathetic nervous system and the other hormone regulators to slow down a little, and tells the parasympathetic nervous system to stop slacking and come a little more into the picture. Temporarily, but only temporarily, it is bringing mind and body back to the balancing systems of healthy stress. But if you sit back at this stage and do nothing further to correct the source of the stress you will achieve very little, and run the risk of dependence on the pills. You will not like the sound of this because it means the ball is back in your court again. You thought you had got rid of it in Chapter 5 after you had first of all examined why you were under stress and then tried to remove it. But you can never entirely take away personal responsibility for coping with stress. If you feel better on tranquillizers you can look at your problems again in a new light and see a way ahead. We are living at a time when drug treatment for harmful stress is criticized because it is claimed to obscure the real problems, but this will only happen if they are taken for an unnecessarily long period. At first they often expose or clarify the problems by changing you from being frightened and unsettled to a state of temporary calm. If you use this breathing space wisely you will have no difficulty in stopping the tranquillizers when the time comes (provided that they are not barbiturates or alcohol).

There are many ways in which your doctor can respond to your cry for help and I have only dealt with the most common. Perhaps we need reminding just how common are prescriptions for tranquillizers, averaging nearly one per person per year in most countries, and costing many millions of pounds. Your doctor can choose any of the other forms of treatment described elsewhere in this book but it will take more time than giving a tranquillizer and may also need special skills that not every doctor possesses. At present doctors are under attack for over-prescribing tranquillizers and sedatives but it is unfair that they should receive all the blame. Many patients feel cheated if they do not come out of a medical interview with a prescription of some sort, and these attitudes put pressure on doctors to give prescriptions, sometimes against their better judgement.

So if you go to your doctor for help with stress you should know what to expect. The likeliest outcome is a prescription for a tablet or medicine and some reassurance. You are going to him in a crisis and he is giving first aid, but seldom more. If he knows you well he may give you a great deal more than reassurance and give helpful advice on combating your particular stress. He may also investigate aspects of physical disease or refer you for specialized psychiatric treatment. Although few of the treatments he has available are particularly good at relieving stress in the long run, they are probably the most predictably effective in the short term. Doctors can now guarantee to reduce nervous tension and if they choose not to give you such treatment it is because of its long-term dangers rather than incompetence or spite. The reasons for different personalities reading this chapter early or late in the book is related to this issue. The Alphas and Gammas have read it early because they are less responsive to treatments described in other chapters and may need the help of tranquillizers during later therapy. I am also unhappy about them resorting to unofficial tranquillizers such as alcohol as a way of relieving their stress, because these are much more dangerous.

Once the immediate pains of stress are relieved by medicines the Alphas should move on to Chapter 10 and the Gammas to Chapter 9. It is impossible to predict when the move from first-aid to more fundamental treatments should take place, because reactions to stress differ so much, but tranquillizers and other pills alone should seldom be taken for more than a few months. Nervous tension is relieved within hours or days but it may take several weeks before depressive illness is brought under control. But once first aid has worked it is time for you to take over the responsibility for dealing with your stress again and not leave it in the hands of the doctor. It is the people who regard medical treatment as the only way of coping with stress who are the ones who will suffer most and are liable to stay on tablets indefinitely. This would not matter if it solved their stressful problems but it often makes them persist. The square peg remains in the round hole but sits a fraction more comfortably because it is lubricated by medicine. The desire to leave the round hole for a square one or convert your existing hole into a better shape gradually dies through apathy and the stress goes on and on.

Most of you will be moving on to other forms of treatment and can put the policy of personal responsibility for stress into effect. The Etas and Epsilons should go to Chapter 10 and the Deltas to Chapter 8. This leaves us with our placid Betas and dependent Zetas, who will be reading this chapter last. They do so for different reasons. The Betas, provided they have been honest in completing their questionnaires and are really placid types, will rarely get to the crisis stage of stress when a visit to the doctor is necessary. If they ever do, the stress has to be excessively severe, such as that endured by the naval rating in the battleship described at the beginning of this book. We are fortunate in peace-time that few stresses of this severity last long, so a tranquillizer is only necessary for a very short period. I therefore feel quite confident that a single prescription will be enough. After this the placid Beta's great resources of healthy stress will take over and the problem will be under control.

Our dependent Zetas come to this chapter last because they are the most susceptible to discarding personal responsibility for stress. They have the tendency to hand over all the difficult problems of life to other people to solve, and occupy themselves with the easy ones. They are only too happy to visit the doctor at the first sign of harmful stress because this will absolve them from doing something positive themselves to overcome it. It will also allow them to blame the doctor if the treatment is not successful. Dependent types are very good at making other people feel guilty for not trying hard enough, and usually get more attention and concern than other folk. If tranquillizers or other pills are successful in making them feel better, they all too frequently sit back and think there is nothing more to be done (apart from getting repeat prescriptions regularly). Any chronic consumer of pills can make out he is an invalid, and dependent types are better than most at this exercise. They are treated as though they are physically and mentally unfit and protected from many of the demands of life. But in the long term they will not do themselves any good and probably create more harmful stress in those about them.

Even if the doctor recognizes the dangers of drug therapy there remain other problems. Zetas are not only likely to become dependent on pills, but also on people. They are amongst the persistent visitors to doctors' surgeries whether or not they have any true illness. They can develop a strong relationship with their doctor which can get out of control. The relationship is almost all one way, basically selfish and quite unhealthy. The patient forgets that he or she is only one of many hundreds treated by the doctor and will often ask for advice about the most trivial problems and at most unsocial hours. Abnormal dependence has to be dealt with in treatment but I hope that Zetas will have tried other ways of overcoming stress first with therapists who have more time and special skills in turning it to the advantage of treatment. I know this may sound harsh language to those who are only a short way along the road to dependence but if I have scared you off tranquillizers it will have done some good.

8

Breaking Bad Habits

Harmful stress, as I have emphasized earlier, is uncompensated stress. All the anti-stress devices are called into action but fail to get the mind and body back into balance. We commonly assume that the stress goes on affecting us because of things going on around us, and are reluctant to consider whether we ourselves might be contributing in some way. In the last twenty years it has been realized that the way we behave in response to stress has a great deal to do with its persistence. To use the jargon of feedback again, we positively reinforce stress in our attempts to control it. In more homely language, we get into bad habits.

Breaking the bad habits of illness is really the province of psychologists, because they are trained in the theory and practice of normal and abnormal behaviour. Psychologists, unlike psychiatrists, are not trained in medicine, and it is not always easy to seek their advice directly. It is possible for doctors to refer people to psychologists if a problem is considered to be in their field but it is often difficult for a patient to seek a psychologist's help directly. But this chapter is concerned with advances in the treatment of harmful stress that have come from the research of psychologists, and much of it is easily available. Many forms of relaxation training have been devised by psychologists from first principles and we have already come across these in an earlier chapter. Relaxation training is a form of behaviour therapy although you may think it odd that feeling tense is a form of behaviour.

85

But if we consider what happens to tension in stress it is very much a behaviour. When we feel tense our muscles are tight and knotted and we cannot help noticing the difference from when we are relaxed. The feeling of tension is unpleasant and often distracts us from other things that we should be doing. Like the nagging pain of a toothache it reminds us that all is not well, and naturally makes us feel a little anxious. But when we feel anxious we have an increase in blood flow to the muscles, so the tension increases. Our positive feedback cycle has started. Each time we worry about our muscular tension it gets worse, so there is more worry and still more tension. Relaxation training (and similar techniques) breaks into this cycle and, if successful, prevents it from getting out of control. It replaces it with a new cycle, the negative feedback of healthy stress. If we are able to bring on muscle relaxation at will whenever we feel tense the cycle of muscle relaxation – mental relaxation – further muscle relaxation is developed.

Behaviour depends on feedback of many different kinds. If we do something and are rewarded for it we are more likely to repeat that behaviour than if we are punished. But although we tend to accept this for parts of behaviour that involve our whole beings, we have been less inclined to accept it for parts of the body. But psychologists have taken it even further. They have suggested that even the activities of the autonomic nervous system can be regarded as behaviour which can be under conscious control. Autonomic systems are by definition self-regulating, and the idea that we can control the actions of our parasympathetic and sympathetic nervous systems is a revolutionary one. Although it has not been confirmed it has led to an interesting new treatment for stress called biofeedback.

If you have looked into ways of treating stress you

have probably heard of biofeedback, because it is widely advertised for this purpose. Many of the advertisements are misleading because they give the impression that stress can be measured on an instrument and you can tell your level of stress by checking the instrument reading. Nothing in the world of stress is as simple as this and to understand biofeedback we need to know the theory behind it. It is based on the idea that all the bodily reactions to stress described in Chapter 2 are potentially under our own control, provided we use the right techniques. Once they are brought under control the positive feedback cycle we have just described with muscle tension is broken and harmful stress eliminated. The techniques of yoga and relaxation we talked about earlier also have the same aim, but they concentrate mainly on the mental side of the cycle. Where biofeedback differs is that with the aid of special instruments you can get a much better idea of how your body is reacting to stress than if you just rely on your senses. With this extra information you can learn better control of your body.

Let us look at an example. We noted earlier that when we get anxious we sweat more than usual, particularly on the palms and soles. The amount we sweat can be measured by an instrument which records how much resistance there is in the skin to the passage of a small electrical current. When we sweat we produce a salty solution which lowers the resistance; when our skin is dry the resistance is raised. The instrument is called a psychogalvanometer; it sounds more impressive than a sweat recorder. The resistance can be shown on a dial or converted to a noise. This is biofeedback. The 'bio' part shows that the instrument measures a biological function, and feedback we already know well. None of this is of value to us unless we can reduce the amount of sweating by getting the feedback. There is reasonable evidence that this can be done, although it is not cast iron. It would be too complicated to go into all the arguments for and against controlling simple biological functions by bio-feedback but let us assume for the time being that we can. Does this mean there should be psychogalva-nometers in every chemist's shop and department store, so that passers-by can get an instant stress reading? And when we feel stress is harming us should we buy a personal psychogalvanometer to learn how to bring our sweating under control? No. The simple idea that because sweating is increased in stress, therefore sweating measures stress, is wrong. First of all there are many other reasons for sweating apart from stressful ones. When the weather is hot and humid we sweat more and after vigorous exercise we also sweat profusely. This does not mean we all get nervous when we exercise, or the Olympic Games would be the Panic Games, and Eskimos would never get anxious. But the second reason is even more damaging to this idea. Although if we compared the amount of sweating in a hundred people under stress with a hundred calm people we would find more sweating on average in the stressful group, there would be many individuals in the stress group who had lower sweating than the sweatiest people in the calm group. I am sure this fits in with your own experience. You must know at least a few placid sweaty people, and a few nervous ones with dry skin. A dry-skinned nervous person under very severe stress will record a low stress reading on a psychogalvanometer and even if he reduces his stress successfully his reading will stay low.

The only people who may find biofeedback with a psychogalvanometer helpful are those whose sweating is closely linked to their general reaction to stress, but these are a minority. Although psychogalvanometers are relatively cheap it is not a wise investment to buy one before knowing whether you are in the small group who are likely to respond. Of course there are more instruments available which measure the function of other parts of the body. All of them involve sticking metal discs or pads to the skin close to the part of the body concerned. Heart rate and muscle tension are most commonly measured and even brain waves can be recorded and played back to the person through a microphone. The people who seem to be helped most by biofeedback are those who show harmful stress as muscle tension and pains, headaches and migraine. Provided that the right group of muscles is chosen and that when they are relaxed the symptoms get less, the technique can be most effective. The person concentrates on reducing tension in the muscles. If he is successful the feedback, usually in the form of clicks or a continuous sound, gets less. Even a tiny reduction in tension is picked up and so the person can work at a wide range of manoeuvres to find which is the best at reducing the symptoms.

You will recognize many similarities between biofeedback, yoga and other forms of relaxation training. Biofeedback is like a Western equivalent of yoga. Both have the same aim, to reduce tension and promote inner tranquillity, but whereas yoga and meditation rely on mystical incantations and instructions, biofeedback relies on an idol of the Western world, a machine which tells us about quantity more than quality. One belongs to religion, the other to science, but they share more than they like to admit. If you choose biofeedback, and you will note from the chapter order that I recommend yoga and similar techniques first (mainly because they are less expensive), then it is wise to consult a psychologist first. Biofeedback is just one way of unlearning the bad habits of harmful stress and there may be others that are suitable for your particular problem. If you can say of your problem, 'I know what I ought to be doing but somehow cannot seem to do it right,' then you could be in this category. The chances are that something you do to reduce the stress is increasing it and that a programme designed to unlearn this harmful response may get rid of the stress. The wrong response can vary from fat people who eat much more after an argument because it makes them feel better, to nervous people with unreasonable fears (phobias) who avoid all the places that bring on the fears and thereby make them worse. Examples could fill a whole book but most of them show the same pattern. Some way of coping is learnt which seems to work immediately but over a long period it makes the problem worse. The trouble is that people are reluctant to give up the ways that seem to work in the short term because the alternative may temporarily make them feel worse. If you take an alcoholic drink whenever you feel tense you will usually feel better afterwards, but when the effect of the alcohol has worn off it is a different story. At a more complex level, if you respond to an argument with your husband or wife by saying nothing for three days, it will certainly avoid further argument immediately but could cause long-term damage to the marriage. The tendency for us to do those things that we are rewarded for and stop doing other things that produce no immediate benefit depends on laws of conditioning. Where a psychologist can help is by setting up new rewards and punishments to replace the ones that are failing to resolve the stress. So the 'silent treatment' after an argument between husband and wife is replaced by an agreement for both parties to talk through the difficulties till they are sorted out.

Many people find it hard to believe that this type of approach is of any value in treating stress. So much of it appears to be common sense, so why should a specialist's help be needed? Help would not be needed if our heads always ruled our hearts, and we always did the rational sensible thing. But we are often led by our emotions to do things which we seem powerless to prevent. I have asked the ambitious, worrying, fussy and suspicious personality types to read this chapter earlier than others because these types are more likely to be conditioned than other types. To put it another way, they are more likely to develop bad habits. Of course the type of conditioning varies tremendously. The ambitious types are heavily conditioned by success, so everything they do which leads to material success is encouraged even if it destroys mind and body in the process. The psychologist can show that success can be obtained just as easily by delegating more work and spending less time on it, without the damaging punishment of stress. The worrying types are conditioned by fear. By trying to avoid anxiety in life they find it everywhere, and eventually it becomes part of them. Real fears are replaced by imagined ones; round every corner there is a tiger waiting to pounce. By teaching mastery of anxiety through relaxation techniques, biofeedback and self-assertion, these types can improve their self-confidence and prevent their surroundings from dictating their actions. They will still be worriers but are no longer imprisoned by anxiety. Our fussy types are similar in some ways. They organize their lives along rigid tramlines and get put out by change that is in any way out of the ordinary. They get conditioned into thinking that no change can be for the better and continue along their well-worn grooves when everyone else has adapted long ago. But we have all to be prepared for rapid and unexpected changes in life. Our fussy types surrounded by stability often cope extremely badly with bereavement. If we have been very close to a relative or friend for many years and he or she dies suddenly, a tremendous readjustment is needed. We have to reconstruct our lives, but if the central pillar has been taken away it is difficult to stop the whole house falling down. Most of us get by with support from other relatives, through religious belief or by throwing ourselves wholeheartedly into something quite new. But our fussy types with their set routines find this extremely difficult, and often take to ruminating about the dead person and continuing their lives in exactly the same manner as before. The first stress is not resolved and gradually becomes harmful stress because the necessary rebuilding has not been done. With psychological help this pattern can be avoided, but if it gets out of control the stress will eventually surface as severe depressive illness.

Suspicious types are conditioned by mistrust and jealousy and need strong secure relationships. But give them a chink of suspicion to work on and they will prise it wide open. A casual remark about liking another person will be interpreted as an indication of a secret affair that has been going on for months or years. Unfortunately once a pattern of mistrust has developed it is almost impossible to deal with by reason alone. The more the innocent wife denies that she is having an affair, the stronger is the belief of her husband that she must be having one, for otherwise why would she deny it so vehemently. If she chooses to be offhand about it the jealousy is still reinforced, for then she is accused of hiding something. The psychologist has to start on a completely new tack. He can teach techniques which avoid rumination and anxiety and alleviate suspicion indirectly.

It is not always necessary to have special help in breaking bad habits. By reading this chapter you may have identified some bad habits of your own and can see ways of getting them changed. Your problems and goals will be the same but you will realize that you have not been successful in getting rid of the stress because of a persistently inappropriate way of going about it. Even if you do not think the way you always use to cope with the problem is wrong it would do you no harm to try a different way next time. Bad habits do not disappear on their own. Things you do make them persist or remove them. Doing nothing at all will also allow the habits to die out in time, but it may take many months and the ambitious types for one will not be able to tolerate this. Deconditioning is better but it needs a push to get started. Changing bad habits that have gone on for years is like opening an old door. The first time it is opened it creaks and shudders before yielding to the weight, the hinges need oiling and protest with creaks and groans. But the more the door is opened the easier it is to move until before long no special effort is needed. Look for those hidden doors in your life before deciding that all your habits are good ones.

Alphas should now move to Chapter 10, Betas, Zetas and Etas to Chapter 7, and Gammas and Epsilons to Chapter 9. The carefree Deltas have finished apart from the final chapter. They are the least liable to develop bad habits in the psychological sense, and are much more likely to have problems because they have no habits to keep. An action only becomes a habit if it is repeated and Deltas, in their endless search for variety, will seldom do the same thing twice.

9

Let's Talk About It

We all talk about problems, some much more than others. This chapter is concerned with talking as a form of treatment for harmful stress, and if you have followed the book in the right order you will realize that talking treatments involve specially trained people who have skills which members of your family and close friends do not possess. Of course if they did have them your stress would not have progressed to the stage of asking for special help. Talking treatment is called psychotherapy and the thought of it provokes quite different reactions in our personality types.

Alphas, as we know, never have enough time to do the things they would like to do, and talking is unnecessarily time-consuming for them. The idea of talking as a form of treatment is something that often annoys them intensely. If the talk is in the form of concise advice which can be easily and quickly understood there is less of a problem, but talking vaguely about their difficulties in the hope of understanding them better is quite another matter. They are reading this chapter last because psychotherapy is likely to make their hackles rise, but if everything else has failed it is in their interests to look at it seriously.

Placid Betas are quite happy to talk about problems, provided that the talking makes few demands on them. They adopt the policy that all is going to turn out for the best and there is no point in rushing things. So psychotherapy for them has to be superficial; they will not take kindly to deep probing and questions about their feelings and wishes that force them to think too much. But for most of their problems a superficial approach is well suited as the harmful stress is not likely to last long.

Our worrying Gammas are sympathetic to any treatment that is going to stop them worrying. As they have been anxious all their lives they have plenty of time and this is no object. Above all they would like to know why they are so nervous and whether there is some deep-rooted cause in the long distant past. They will take psychotherapy very seriously and will co-operate well with the therapist. Delta types are also happy to talk about solving the problems of stress. They usually talk easily and well but find more difficulty in persevering with treatment. Their need for variety makes them search for rapid solutions rather than follow a steady course taking up to several months. But if they are prepared to stay the course they can be helped, which is why they are reading this chapter at an early stage.

Suspicious Epsilons are in two minds about psychotherapy. They often need to discuss their difficulties but they do not like disclosing confidential details about themselves. They will only talk openly when they have complete trust in the therapist. They are also highly sensitive people and do not take criticism well, so discussing ways of overcoming stress requires patience and tact as well as understanding. But dependent Zetas are chatterboxes. They positively relish the chance to talk about their troubles, but although they appear to make great progress it is difficult for them to convert talk into action. They know what they should do and talk often about doing it, but when the time comes they do nothing. So many of their decisions are made for them by other people and they find it hard to take independent action. For them talking is a pleasant interlude which all too often ends with a new and satisfying relationship but no more.

Fussy Etas share the concern of their fellow Alphas about the value of talk. They are quite happy with simple straightforward advice but do not like the vagueness of talk about themselves. Although they say that they dislike it because it does not lead anywhere, sometimes they are concerned because they are afraid that really fundamental talk about themselves and their lives might completely overturn their elaborately organized lives and leave them with no replacements. Some fussy meticulous people are insecure and use order as a way of protecting themselves, so any threat to that order will mobilize their defences. Etas also try very hard to raise reason above feelings; they look for the logical rational explanation rather than the emotional one, but as so much of harmful stress is concerned with feelings they cannot avoid the subject. Talking may help them a great deal, but many barriers have to be broken down first.

I am not going to pretend that your reaction to talking treatment is necessarily going to fit in with the one attached to your personality type, but you can at least see the wide range of reactions to psychotherapy. Up to now we have only discussed talking in general terms. How can it counteract harmful stress and who should be involved in it? Psychotherapy can be carried out at several different levels. We all use it at its most simple level. Reassuring and comforting people in distress, and listening and commenting on their problems sympathetically are good examples. This can be done without any special understanding or great knowledge of the person in distress. At a deeper level of psychotherapy we need to know something more about the sufferer. What sort of person is he, and what special circumstances have made him react in this way at this time? In answering these questions, it is as though a surface map is made of the person and his surroundings, a map which is unique but which shares many features with others. The therapist should have special knowledge of the type of problem so that he can give constructive advice, advice which the sufferer is unlikely to have received from elsewhere. For this type of psychotherapy it is important to go to the right person. If harmful stress is shown in marriage it is reasonable to consult a marriage guidance counsellor. Such counsellors are specially trained in understanding and advising about marital problems; they know from experience the features that make personalities clash together and prevent difficulties from being resolved. So they are not advising in a vacuum; they have seen problems like this before and can see solutions to them even if you cannot. If a marital stress problem is in the sexual sphere, such as impotence, frigidity or premature ejaculation, further help may be needed, possibly from psychological treatments described earlier, which look on these as bad habits which require retraining. Outside marital problems marriage guidance counsellors are not so effective because their experience of other difficulties is less; they do not recognize the problem 'maps' presented to them so solutions are not so easy.

If the harmful stress is related to problems of guilt, or with life making no sense and having no meaning, then, depending on your religious convictions, the church may be the place to go for your psychotherapy. It may sound strange to refer to religious communication in such a way, but a great deal of psychotherapy is involved. The minister or priest has special knowledge of you and your type of problem and can point the way to a solution. The confession of sin is a most potent form of therapy and is imitated by doctors practising psychotherapy. Wiping the slate clean and starting afresh is an excellent way of dealing with harmful stress.

If the stress is bound up with the circumstances of our

day to day living it may be appropriate to seek the help of a social worker. Although many think of social workers as just giving advice about housing and social security problems, or rescuing those who are down and out, they also have skills in psychotherapy. So in addition to practical advice you may be involved in more deep-seated discussions. Very few of us have problems which are entirely caused by housing, money or job difficulties. We tend to bring problems on ourselves and unfortunately we all too frequently repeat our mistakes when the same circumstances arise in the future. Do not get angry, therefore, at apparent interference by social workers asking questions and making observations on matters which you regard as outside their sphere.

The deeper levels of psychotherapy are usually practised by psychiatrists and psychoanalysts. They regard their task as quite different from that of other talking treatments. They are not concerned with constructing a surface map of the person and his problem but a complete map, including all the deeper layers as well as what is shown on the surface. It is not easy to get to these deeper levels. Therapists probe them by analysing dreams and by other techniques, all of which involve talking, not just for a few minutes, but often for hundreds of hours. The common stereotype of a psychiatrist is that of a mysterious man who talks in a mid-European accent, seldom gives a straight answer to a straight question, and who carries out all his treatment with his patient lying on a couch. If you expect your psychiatrist to be like this you will almost certainly be disappointed, but psychoanalysis is based on this general approach. It is very difficult to recommend when to turn to this type of therapy because it is usually expensive and very time-consuming, and the surface appearance of the problem often tells us very little of what is going on underneath.

In general it is better to consider the psychoanalytical approach only when the harmful stress has become chronic and has resisted all other efforts to remove it.

One obvious question comes up at this point. Can people really change in themselves in order to overcome harmful stress or can they only change their circumstances? Are we really stamped with our personalities for life? We have already seen how Alpha personality types, for example, tend to seek out stress more than others and are more likely to suffer as a consequence. It would solve so many of Alphas' problems if they could all be altered to placid Betas. Sorry, it cannot be done, and the only ray of hope I can offer is to add that if you are less than twenty-five years old you are likely to be still developing your personality and can still alter course a little. But the amount you can change is limited, so do not expect miracles. Far too many people oversimplify their problems of stress and personality by thinking that if they go on a long quest into the depths of their unconscious they will find the gremlin that is the cause of their troubles, which when exposed and destroyed will explain and alter everything. Dazzling insights into ourselves can happen but they do not change our basic personalities. What they are able to do, and this is where psychotherapy in all its forms can help, is to strip off the layers of phoney personality that we all cover ourselves with from time to time. We all protect ourselves to some extent with coatings of façade, and often these are so impressive they appear real. They deceive others so well that we also begin to think they are true. If we fool ourselves in this way without realizing it we are apt to become what we are not, parodies of ourselves in roles that others would like us to play but which are not our true selves. When you see people about you who seem to have undergone a transformation in personality there is unlikely to have been any basic change. They have either peeled off their phoney costumes or climbed into new ones, but eventually the real personality will show through again.

So deep psychotherapy may help us to understand ourselves better so that what we do and how we feel makes more sense, but it is rarely going to dramatically change us. How it is going to help cannot be predicted at the outset and no one is going to be able to make any definite predictions or give guarantees. An ideal response to treatment can be the acceptance of yourself as you are in such a way that harmful mental stress is resolved. All those doubts about insecurity and fear of the future disappear because you are no longer running away from yourself. At a different level your attitudes can change so that the ideal job for which you have been striving, or the girlfriend who is the only possible wife for you, no longer seem so important, and the harmful stress that has resulted from them can be eliminated. So do not be disheartened; although personalities cannot change, attitudes can, and it is our attitudes that govern much of our daily lives; all those trivial things that do not seem much on their own but which take up most of our time.

Deltas, Gammas and Zetas should now proceed to Chapter 10, Betas to Chapter 8, and Epsilons to Chapter 7. Alphas and Etas have completed their tour and need only to read the final chapter.

10

Keeping Fit

People have odd notions about keeping fit. Many think they are fit if they feel well and have no signs of ill-health, but if asked to run a hundred yards will be unable to manage more than twenty. They protest that successful running needs super fitness requiring special training and should not be expected of the man in the street. Others think of fitness as the muscular strength of the body beautiful, and try to mimic Charles Atlas and Mr Universe by strenuous body-building exercises using chest expanders and bar bells. Yet others think physical fitness can only be achieved by professionals or full-time sportsmen and it is pointless for part-timers to get involved. There are also some funny ideas about women and fitness. Men are often expected to spend part of their day in some physical activity, which may be as strenuous as a work-out in a gym or as mild as exercising the family dog, but women are denied the same right. There is no good reason for this attitude, which is based on prejudice. Women have the same right to be fit as men, and this is not going to be achieved just by pushing a vacuum cleaner round the carpet, hanging the washing on the line, and the other hundred and one domestic chores that too many men expect women to do while they carry out their programmed fitness exercises.

What has fitness got to do with harmful stress? To answer this we come back to the idea of balance between mind and body. We noted earlier that we live in an era of specialization. Society forces us into spending much of our time using only the skills for which we have been trained. Because of increasing automation very few of these skills involve healthy exercise. Even the farm worker and manual labourer, who get much more healthy exercise in their work than the rest of us, have many machines to do the jobs which their predecessors were forced to do with their bare hands. The rest of us are denied even a modicum of exercise in our work. We sit at desks in offices exercising no part of our bodies below the neck, so it is not surprising that the rest of our frames cry out for activity and fall into disrepair and disease if it is not received. We abuse our bodies still more by many of our habits. Breathing the polluted air of cigars and cigarettes, or the smoke and dust of congested cities and industrial plants, damages our lungs and makes us less able to satisfy the demands of exercise. We eat too much of the wrong foods, stuffing ourselves with fats and carbohydrates rather than extra protein. The carbohydrates in sweet and starchy foods are excellent for giving rapid energy but if we do not take up the offer and exercise our bodies it is converted to fat, adding yet another roll to the expanding waistline. It is all too easy in these days of refined and concentrated foods to eat more than the 2,500 calories a day that most of us can get by on quite happily. And of course if we go beyond this we get fat and find exercising even more of a bind. Fat people are sluggish and need fewer calories than thin ones, so they find it harder than most to lose weight. All too frequently they give up and decide they are 'naturally' overweight and point to some distant relative who was over twenty stone yet was hale and hearty till death at an advanced age. The trouble is that when our bodies run to seed in this way we have very little reserves to call upon when put under stress. When discussing conscious healthy stress early in this book we noted that when our sympathetic nervous systems are stimulated we put our bodies and minds temporarily out of balance, and the fitter we are the more rapidly we return to normal. For those who are unfit it may take a whole day to shake off the effects, but there can be even worse results. An over-weight man with furred-up arteries and an inefficient heart has so little in reserve that even the excitement of watching a comedy show or sport on television can prove to be too demanding – with fatal consequences.

Keeping fit not only protects us from stress damaging our bodies but also aids our mental mechanisms. Sitting in a chair all day may appear to be physically relaxing but it is a marvellous promoter of tension. All of us get frustrated and angry from time to time, Alpha and Delta types more than others, but we have to suppress the natural physical consequences of these feelings. We cannot club the boss over the head when he upsets us or run into the distance when he approaches with a threaten-ing scowl. But if we can get rid of these frustrations later such as by hitting a punchball vigorously while ima-gining that it has just the same size, shape and sense as the boss's head, or by running five miles, we shall feel better, and much more relaxed.

So keeping fit both protects us from future stress and helps us to cope with current stress. The best way of keeping fit is to exercise the whole body so that all parts build up reserves and become more efficient. Exercise in the form of running, swimming, walking or cycling is therefore a great deal better than weight-lifting, press-ups and all forms of exercise which take place while stand-ing still. This may annoy those who equate physical fit-ness with muscular prowess, as a well-trained fit person is not particularly muscular in appearance although he has a higher proportion of muscle to other tissues than an unfit person. Because he has no excess fat a fit athlete may even be described as scrawny or weedy, but do not be put off by his appearance for he has tremendous reserves.

What is the best way of keeping fit? There is no best way and your choice will depend on your personality type. The important thing is that whatever form of exercise you take, it should involve your whole body and be intense enough to increase your heart rate and make you a little breathless. By doing this you are training your body to be more efficient so that the next time you do the same exercise you will be less breathless and recover more rapidly.

Alpha types have little time for physical fitness but they are good at responding to a challenge. They like to be able to measure progress in exact terms, not just in the way they feel. It is best for them to set aside a defined period each day from their busy timetables in order to take their exercise. Their exercise should have a goal, an achievement that can be bettered with increasing fitness. A points system such as the one developed by Dr Kenneth Cooper and described in his book *Aerobics* is ideal for Alphas. The system can be used for running, stationary running, swimming, cycling, walking and sports such as squash and basketball, and includes programmes for reaching and maintaining fitness. It will also help Alphas if they cut down on undesirable habits which hinder fitness. The stresses that they seek out in their lives make them more likely than others to be tobacco smokers. They will soon realize that their fitness programme is much easier to attain if they cut down their smoking or stop altogether. Once the tar is cleared out of their lungs they will have no desire to return to the habit.

Beta types hate the idea of fitness programmes. Their naturally placid temperaments cannot see any point in doing unnecessary exercise to get fit and they would not have the persistence to keep up a points system. They are best advised to take their exercise in a more practical way. Their natural laziness inclines them to take the easiest way out of any problem and they rely too much on machines to do work for them. But if they live only a mile or two from their place of work they can easily walk instead of taking the car. Better still, they can cycle, which is a marvellous way of keeping fit. Instead of using the motor mower on the lawn they can root out that old hand mower that has not been used for years. Of course it takes more effort but the results are much more satisfying. Most of these changes will take a little longer than the lazy alternatives, but as Betas are not too concerned about time this should not be a problem.

Betas also tend to run to fat, as they enjoy their food and are less active than other types. The chief reason I have asked Betas to read this chapter at an early stage is that sloth and over-eating are the habits that are most likely to cause harmful stress in them. If they are overweight and increase their exercise they are tempted to think that nothing more is necessary. But exercise has to be long and strenuous to lose even a few pounds in weight and some form of reducing diet will probably be needed as well. There are dozens of dieting techniques and I am not going to go into detail about them. Almost without exception they require a drastic reduction in the amount of carbohydrate in the diet. All of them, if followed accurately, will lead to the body being temporarily starved of food. When this happens, the body's own food stores of fat will be mobilized and burnt to make energy. Obviously during this process you are going to feel hungry, and often ravenous. The temptation to nibble between meals or slightly exceed the diet quota becomes very strong. If you succumb to it you may not lose weight but it is dishonest to conclude that the diet has failed and that you stay fat no matter how much you eat.

Nervous Gammas often question whether physical fitness is going to help their problems as these are mainly in the mental sphere. They have forgotten those times in the past when they had just finished some long or vigorous exercise, whether in sport or another recreation such as fell walking, rambling or even digging the garden. The feeling of relaxation that follows is not just the absence of tension from the hard worked muscles but a mental peace that sweeps over and replaces the worries of the day. Good exercise can be an excellent tranquillizer and makes you healthier into the bargain. Just think what a relief it must be for the bodies of Gamma types to have healthy exercise. Their sympathetic nervous systems are always being stimulated for action, like runners in their blocks waiting for the starter's pistol to fire, but far too often they fail to act, paralysed in painful anticipation for the next stress to appear. If you are a Gamma type and cannot relax with techniques such as yoga and auto-hypnosis, try them again after a period of exercise such as running or swimming. You will find them to be much more effective.

Carefree Deltas need a range of exercises rather than concentrating on one and improving performance. Their need for variety leads them into unusual hobbies and often gives scope for exercise. Again the same points apply. If the exercise is sufficiently strenuous to produce breathlessness and increase heart rate it is valuable and healthy, whether it is obtained by cycling penny-farthings, underwater swimming with breathing apparatus or abseiling down cliffs. There is a tendency for Delta types to drink more alcohol than other types and if this becomes excessive it will not help their physical fitness. If you take a close look at the regular drinkers at your local pub, how many of them do you think could run a mile without feeling shattered? Drink has a gradual effect on fitness which takes place long before it does permanent damage to the stomach and liver, and its consumption needs to be kept under control.

Epsilons and Zetas have opposing personalities and need to take different forms of exercise. Epsilons are naturally solitary and prefer to exercise alone. Cross-country running is ideal for them. It allows them to take on the world alone. The cross-country runner is the complete individual; he owes nothing to others and has to rely entirely on his own resources. Even in training he can work alone. Zetas are gregarious and need people, and their exercise is much more pleasant when carried out in groups. One possible reason for the upsurge of interest in jogging is that it can be a group enterprise. The strain of competitive running is absent and the pace is such that the whole family can take part. Sports that involve groups such as doubles tennis and squash are also liked by Zetas. There is time to talk between points and playing in a team takes away the personal responsibility of playing alone. Solitary exercise is not worth exploring by Zetas; it has too many disadvantages to be taken seriously.

Etas are fussy and methodical and, like most of their life's activities, exercise is taken seriously. It needs planning and organization, and will usually be incorporated into a ritual, as predictable as the morning visit to the lavatory to move the bowels. The ritual can vary from person to person but once it has become established it sticks. A run before breakfast, a walk with the dog in the evening, a 100 yard swim every Tuesday and Thursday, a game of handball or squash every Friday, are just a few examples. Others may make fun of these rituals but Etas are much better at maintaining fitness because of them.

The important thing is to make sure that at least one exercise ritual is included in the repertoire.

Alphas, Betas and Etas should now move on to Chapter 9, Deltas to Chapter 7 and Zetas to Chapter 8. Gammas and Epsilons have completed their tortuous route and can finish by reading the last chapter. Whatever the nature of their stress and personalities, I hope that all types now realize the value of positive physical fitness, as opposed to just absence of ill-health, in fighting the effects of harmful stress.

II

Putting Stress in Perspective

'Gentle reader, we are together again.' Writers from yesteryear were kind to their readers, and reassured and coddled them along their book journeys with such phrases. I cannot make claim to the same generosity, but I hope that your tour has been fruitful. Whether you are suffering from stress or reading out of curiosity I think you will have seen the reasons for reading the last five chapters in an odd order. As stress is a personal reaction to change it is pointless giving the same advice to everyone who is suffering harmful stress. I have picked out personality as the key factor in deciding the best approach but you will have also noticed many others – the length and severity of the stress, whether it shows in the mental or physical sphere and whether it follows from problems in relationships or from things about us. In this final chapter we should put all these in perspective.

First I should like to add a final word on personality. Each of us has an ideal level of stress which satisfies us. Below this level we get bored and above it we feel under strain. You will have guessed already that different personalities have different ideal levels of stress. Driving Alphas have the highest levels and Betas the lowest; Gammas and Epsilons have moderately low levels, Zetas and Etas moderately high ones, and Deltas a little higher still. These are not necessarily the levels of stress they encounter in their daily lives, and Gammas in particular would like their stress levels to be much less. These ideal levels indicate the amount of change in their lives and surroundings that each personality type would settle for in the absence of any other considerations. So you can see at a glance that it is impossible for all our personality types to be satisfied in the same situation. The aim is to ensure that once in or near the ideal stress levels, all stress is healthy stress.

If you feel that the type of personality decided by your scores on the questionnaire was quite wrong then you may have been dissatisfied with the advice that I have given. I can understand your feelings and agree that it would be silly to assume that the questionnaire is right and you are wrong. We all have a mixture of personality features and only a few have one dominant characteristic that shows in all aspects of their lives. If your highest score on the questionnaire was 20 points or less no one personality feature is dominant and you have an even mixture. A maximum score of 25 or more suggests that you really do have the appropriate personality type. If it disagrees with your own assessment try asking someone else whom you know well enough to give a frank and honest opinion. You may be surprised at their answers. We all have ideas of the people we should like to be, and it is all too easy for us to pretend we have some or all of these features in our own personalities. Most of us would like to think that we have a good proportion of the placid Beta features in our personalities and very little of the solitary and suspicious Epsilon ones. If the results of the questionnaire tell you otherwise ask yourself whether you have admitted the existence of all the skeletons in your personality cupboard before you blame the questionnaire. This is important because it can be a great help in deciding on the cause of a particular stress. For example if you feel dissatisfied and mentally tense for no apparent reason as everything in your life is settled and serene, the cause may be that you are basically an Alpha type who is understimulated. You may laugh at the suggestion that you are driving and ambitious because nothing you have done to date suggests these qualities. But there is a tiger inside you waiting to get out when you give it the opportunity.

If your maximum score on the questionnaire was between 21 and 25 points you probably have predominance of the personality type indicated by the score but other features are also important. It is quite possible to get high scores on apparently contradictory features such as Alpha and Beta or Zeta and Epsilon characteristics, in which case the overall personality is a fairly balanced one.

If you are seriously troubled by stress it is going to take a great deal more than reading this book to overcome it. At least I trust I have given you an idea how to go about the task. Battles are lost and won as much through tactics and strategy as through courage and fighting skill. Of course you may have given up the battle against stress altogether, in which case I hope I have given you new heart.

For others who have been troubled by harmful stress in the past but are now free, and those who have yet to deal with its unpleasant features, I hope you can see the value of the phrase 'prevention is better than cure'. Although we have seen that stress is not a disease in itself, it lies behind many forms of illness, and doctors all agree that they are not very good at curing these illnesses. This does not mean they cannot help, but curing means removing the problem entirely so that not even a mark is left. Harmful stress has a habit of making indelible marks which cannot be removed, and even partial removal involves a lot of effort. It is so much better to prevent harmful stress from developing. Again and again we come back to the concept of balance, which is at the core of all healthy stress. If our autonomic nervous systems can keep balance so well, surely our conscious nervous systems should be able to do the same. The trouble is that the rules are almost too easy. We have heard them so often we disregard them. We need to keep a balance between work and play, activity and rest, social contacts and isolation, emotions and intellect, between noise and quiet and many other opposing forces. As we have seen, the points of balance vary from one to another but must be present somewhere. No one is going to remain well without some physical activity and even the most isolated hermit needs some contact with his fellow man.

One of the conclusions reached by our visitor from outer space at the beginning of this book was that stress was a scapegoat of our society. Unfortunately I think there is some truth in this, but if we are aware of the danger it can be eliminated. We live in an age in which an explanation is demanded for every happening, and more and more answers are forthcoming. But we shall never have all the answers and many things will remain inexplicable. Rather than admit this, or continue to look for the answer, people can put it all down to stress. As stress can change itself into any shape at will, it will obviously fit the demands of any situation, but all too often it is an explanation in a vacuum. I am sure that reading this book has shown the futility of blaming stress for unpleasant events, feelings or illnesses and doing nothing further about it. The recognition of stress is the beginning of a problem, not the end, and although the way towards a solution, like your route through this book, may be a tortuous one, it is worth the journey.

Index

Overcoming Common Problems Series

For a full list of titles please contact
Sheldon Press, Marylebone Road, London NW1 4DU

Beating Job Burnout
DR DONALD SCOTT

Beating the Blues
SUSAN TANNER AND JILLIAN
BALL

Being the Boss
STEPHEN FITZSIMON

Birth Over Thirty
SHEILA KITZINGER

Body Language
How to read others' thoughts by their
gestures
ALLAN PEASE

Bodypower
DR VERNON COLEMAN

Bodysense
DR VERNON COLEMAN

Calm Down
How to cope with frustration and anger
DR PAUL HAUCK

Changing Course
How to take charge of your career
SUE DYSON AND STEPHEN HOARE

Comfort for Depression
JANET HORWOOD

Complete Public Speaker
GYLES BRANDRETH

**Coping Successfully with Your Child's
Asthma**
DR PAUL CARSON

**Coping Successfully with Your Hyperactive
Child**
DR PAUL CARSON

**Coping Successfully with Your Irritable
Bowel**
ROSEMARY NICOL

Coping with Anxiety and Depression
SHIRLEY TRICKETT

Coping with Blushing
DR ROBERT EDELMANN

Coping with Cot Death
SARAH MURPHY

Coping with Depression and Elation
DR PATRICK McKEON

Coping with Stress
DR GEORGIA WITKIN-LANOIL

Coping with Suicide
DR DONALD SCOTT

Coping with Thrush
CAROLINE CLAYTON

Curing Arthritis – The Drug-Free Way
MARGARET HILLS

Curing Arthritis Diet Book
MARGARET HILLS

**Curing Coughs, Colds and Flu – The
Drug-Free Way**
MARGARET HILLS

Curing Illness – The Drug-Free Way
MARGARET HILLS

Depression
DR PAUL HAUCK

Divorce and Separation
ANGELA WILLANS

Don't Blame Me!
How to stop blaming yourself
and other people
TONY GOUGH

The Epilepsy Handbook
SHELAGH McGOVERN

**Everything You Need to Know about
Adoption**
MAGGIE JONES

**Everything You Need to Know about
Contact Lenses**
DR ROBERT YOUNGSON

**Everything You Need to Know about
Osteoporosis**
ROSEMARY NICOL

Overcoming Common Problems Series

Over**c**oming  **S**eries